D0915968

HOW DOES IT FEEL TO BE BLIND ?

The Psychodynamics
of Visual Impairment
by
Paul J. Schulz

Published by
Muse-Ed Company
Los Angeles

Muse-Ed Company
14141 Margate Street
Van Nuys, CA 91401

Library of Congress catalog card number: 80-81502

Schulz, Paul J.
 Blindness, Psychology of

ISBN 0-9604434-2-8

Printed in the United States of America

DEDICATIONS

To Sherwin Sloan, M.D., for encouragement and suggestions on
    revision of the book.

To Maurice N. Walsh, M.D., for the many consultations that
    helped shape the direction of my work.

To Carol Johnson for help in editing.

To the many clients who shared their feelings and experiences
    during counseling.

To my colleagues, and

To Peggy, Sylvia, Lisa and Eric.

FOREWORD

To the ophthalmologist, the blindness of a patient may be equivalent to the death of an internist's patient. Indeed, blindness is ophthalmic death. This is why it is difficult for many ophthalmologists, optometrists, or other professionals dealing with visually handicapped patients to continue to care for these patients once they become blind.

Some knowledge of the internal reactions of the newly blind person is essential for those individuals who are concerned with the blind person's medical, social, or economic welfare. By obtaining this knowledge it becomes easier for people to deal with their own emotions in relation to the blind. What could be a painful situation for patient and eye care workers can be turned into a mutually rewarding experience.

Mr. Schulz has elucidated the vast experiences and reactions of the newly blind person in not a sketchy manner, but in a thorough, insightful way. These insights will prove very valuable for the physician, optometrist, social worker, psychologist or any other who may wish to deal with the problems of a blind person.

Sherwin H. Sloan, M.D.
Associate Clinical Professor
of Ophthalmology
UCLA School of Medicine

CONTENTS

Preface
Section I

BLINDNESS   Page

Section II

THE EMOTIONAL REACTION TO THE LOSS OF SIGHT

Section III

FAMILY AND COMMUNITY REACTION

Section IV

ADJUSTMENT TO THE LOSS OF SIGHT

Section V
TREATMENT

SECTION I

THE BLINDNESS EXPERIENCE

CHAPTER 1

THE BLINDNESS EXPERIENCE

Case History — Jim

Jim realized that for some time he had been unable to see well in the dark. Sometimes he stumbled over objects when he came home at night. He also noticed that he did not adapt well to the dark when coming out of a lighted room. Although he tried to convince himself that it wasn't true, he was having great difficulty in reading. He finally had to admit to himself that something was definitely wrong with his eyes. Because he had often been told not to read so much, he blamed himself for what was happening. Many times while he had been reading in the evening, he had read until he could no longer see the print. For this reason, he did not wish to tell his parents what was happening. He felt that if he could only rest his eyes for a few days, his vision would improve.

guilt over cause of blind- ness . . .

Jim had delayed asking for help because he felt his family would be critical. He also had vague feelings of apprehension, but tried to reassure himself with thoughts that a good doctor would soon cure his visual problem. The first ophthalmologist who examined him told him bluntly that there was no cure for his condition and that ultimately he would become totally blind. The doctor also suggested he attend a school for the blind and learn to play some musical instrument. Jim was shocked by this disclosure. He had fully expected to be treated and eventually cured. He also was repelled by the thought of attending a school for the

anxiety . . .

blind. He had once seen a blind man being led awkwardly down some stairs. The look on the man's face as he stumbled filled Jim with pity. At the same time, he was disturbed by a brief feeling of aversion toward the man who was so helpless. Now, when he remembered the experience, he realized that other people could think of him in the same way.

negative feeling toward blindness . . .

Jim was even more upset by the doctor's suggestion for an occupation. His high school work had been average, but then he had never studied very hard. Literature and English had been his favorite subjects and he'd nourished a secret ambition to be a writer. He'd wanted to achieve this goal independently, so he planned to work for a year after his high school graduation, save his money, and then enroll in college.

desire to be independent . . .

Now he felt that he was being told to give up this goal. And to add to this loss, he was being lumped with a lot of blind people. "This doctor doesn't know what he's talking about. I'll get the name of the best specialist in the country and see him. Besides, I'm not really blind; I still have a lot of sight — enough to get around." Thoughts such as these occupied him during this time. He noticed, however, that his sight was deteriorating rapidly. Other doctors examined him. Some told him essentially what the first doctor had reported; others were more vague. Jim, however, maintained the belief that he would find a doctor who could help him. He could not consider the alternative.

denial . . .

unrealistic hope for recovery. . .

Jim graduated from high school, but did not attend any of the social functions such as the prom and other senior activities. Since he could not drive a car, he quit dating. He did not tell his friends about his condition because he dreaded any expressions of pity. And for this reason he dropped out of his old circle of acquaintances.

He tried to hide his poor vision as much as possible — would not carry a cane, and absolutely refused to learn to read braille. Once he was almost struck by a car as he stepped from the sidewalk. The experience was frightening but did not change his behavior. He was often embarrassed when strangers didn't realize he could not see well, such as the time he asked a bus driver, "What bus is this?" and the driver replied sharply, "What's the matter, are you blind? It's right on the front of the bus!" At other times, when he stumbled on a curb or almost fell down stairs that he was unable to see, he felt as though everyone had noticed. While he still retained some sight, he worked in factories as an unskilled assembly line worker. Some employers hired him without being aware of his visual impairment, but when they discovered how little he could see, they usually let him go.

unwillingness to accept identity as blind (identity crisis) . . .

self-consciousness . . .

After three years his vision became so poor he was no longer able to hide the fact. He remained almost continually at home and never seemed to feel really good anymore. Sometimes he felt blue, especially when he thought about the things he used to do that were no longer possible. He could almost feel himself behind the wheel of a car, driving — far and fast.

depressive reaction . . .

fantasy as substitute for reality . . .

Occasionally, a friend would stop by and take him for a drive. Sometimes two or three couples would take him on a beach party, but if no one invited him, he would stay at home rather than ask to join in their activities. Often a friend would make an appointment with him and either show up late or call and cancel the appointment. Jim was always polite in acknowledging these changes of plans, but seethed inwardly when they occurred. Sometimes Jim felt he would like to blow his top when he had waited and been disappointed. However, he was afraid that if he did, he would get no more invitations. Frequently he directed this anger towards his parents, accusing them of not spending enough time with him.

resistance to realistic dependency . . .

suppressed anger . . .

conflict

displaced anger . . .

His parents accepted these outbursts and responded by doing almost everything they could for him. They would lead him from one room to another. When he sat down to eat, they would place his fork in his hand. Far from expecting him to help in household duties, they refused any small offer he made, such as washing dishes or making his bed. Jim gradually drifted into this routine and accepted this passive role.

overprotection contributing to unrealistic dependency . . .

Finally, Jim decided to start writing again. A few of his articles had been published in the high school paper, so he felt he must have some ability. Besides, he had nothing else to do and nothing to lose. Now he experienced practical difficulty. It was nearly impossible to find someone to help him revise his stories. He submitted rough drafts to publishers, and when they were turned down, he blamed the friends who were too busy to help. He told his parents that if he could only see well enough to do his own revision, his stories would be accepted. Blindness was the excuse he most often used for failure. Not only did his parents accept his excuses, but they read him articles describing scientific advances that might help him regain his sight.

blindness as an excuse for failure . . .

family support for unrealistic hope . . .

In spite of what he told his parents, Jim began to doubt his ability. The years of sitting at home had made him feel useless. He was getting nowhere. Yet, whenever a friend suggested that a rehabilitation agency might help him find work, Jim pointed out that he was making progress in his writing, and was quick to mention the difficulties of traveling without sight.

lowered self-esteem . . .

resistance to rehabilitation . . .

Jim had one friend who occasionally took him out for coffee or lunch. They frequented a restaurant where Jim became acquainted with a waitress he liked very much. After several weeks of deliberation, he arranged a double date with his friend. Hesitantly he asked the waitress to go out with him, but she refused. He became acutely depressed. When his mood did not lift, his

acute depressive reaction to seemingly insignificant event . . .

friend suggested he see a psychiatrist.

Jim made progress in psychotherapy, but changing was difficult because he had lived so long with his problems and feelings. In time he was able to mourn his loss and admit that he would never see again. He began to realize that much of his own behavior and attitude were responsible for his isolation. If he was alone, it was because he had withdrawn. If his parents had overprotected him, he had resented it but also had wanted it. Marked improvement began when he admitted he might benefit from special training.

objectivity concerning his condition . . .

decreased resistance to rehabilitation . . .

The change came when he gained insight into the way his anxiety and self-consciousness interfered with what he really wanted to do. Once he realized he need not always be dependent, he became more realistic about his goals. Before he could achieve them, however, he needed training and education. Jim entered a rehabilitation program and learned to travel and take care of his everyday needs. As he became more independent, his self-esteem grew. His anger and frustration diminished as he learned how to do things for himself and no longer had to wait for help.

growing self-esteem from competence . . .

When he completed his rehabilitation program, he enrolled in college. He was now a competent blind person and felt comfortable in this role. Making new friends and renewing former social contacts was easy now that he felt himself to be a worthwhile person. He didn't think of himself as the most popular person on campus, but was pleased with his expanded social life. He had no difficulty in meeting and dating girls who accepted him as he was.

new identity . . .

Eventually, he became confident enough to move into an apartment of his own. Academically he did well, and after completing his education, he obtained a teaching position. With the security of a regular income, he pursued his

original goal and was able to have some of his
articles published.

IS THERE A TYPICAL CASE OF BLINDNESS?

The case of Jim is a description of the way in which one person might react to the loss of sight. His reaction was determined by personality traits, social circumstances, and the physical facts of his visual loss. The various features of the reaction noted in the margin are often present in the experience of others who lose their sight. The frequency with which some of them occur might suggest they are always part of a normal reaction. In terms of a few predominant characteristics this may be true. However, many persons may never experience some of the features described in the case of Jim.

There is, in fact, no typical case of blindness. Severe loss of sight can occur at any period of life. Because the personality and experience of each person is unique, he will react to stress in his own way. Even the manner in which each person loses his sight is distinctive, and thus, his responses will be molded by his own pattern of loss. Furthermore, none of these elements functions independently. They are complexly related, and this complexity contributes to the specific character of the emotional reaction.

The case of Jim is not even the story of one person. It is a composite based on the experience of three young men who lost their sight. It is, however, a factual description in the sense that the events, the reaction, and the resolution did occur. It serves as an illustration of what might happen when an individual loses his sight.

CHAPTER 2

BLINDNESS AND
SEVERE VISUAL IMPAIRMENT

The Popular Concept

The popular concept of blindness is that of a person with absolutely no sight. Many people have an image of a person imprisoned by darkness — stumbling, falling, or groping around in the dark. They imagine a person who is totally inadequate and unable to take care of himself.

Because of this image they are confused when they see a person walking confidently with a white cane or a guide dog. Similarly, they are confused by a person they think of as being blind who looks right at them when he speaks. He seems to find an object he is looking for with no apparent difficulty. If they observe him reading a sign or hear him comment that he is aware of a car or other object near him, they are sure he is a liar or a hypocrite. He is obviously feigning blindness for his own devious reasons.

The difficulty is that most persons have had little or no close contact with a blind or visually impaired person. Their information about "blind" people comes from the infrequent times they have seen a blind man or woman traveling, or from someone who has heard of or knows a blind person.

Blindness is the word commonly used by professionals to describe the condition of the visually impaired persons with whom they work. They use it as a shorthand term to encompass all the degrees and forms of visual limitation. Used in this way, it is not confusing to them because in practice, they are aware of the differences included in the word. But since it does not accurately describe the wide range of visual deficiencies, it is misleading. Furthermore, it coincides with the popular concept of blindness, and thus contributes to general misunderstanding about the condition.

In fact, only a small number of persons classified as blind are totally without sight. Most retain some useful vision. Some have light perception in one or both eyes. Others can see shadows or large objects, such as a car or a building. Still others can see enough to read large print or determine the color of traffic lights when they are close enough. Many can see objects at a distance, but their field vision is severely restricted.

LEGAL BLINDNESS

Severe visual limitation is described by terms such as legal blindness, industrial blindness, functional blindness, visual handicap, or visual impairment. Legal blindness is the most commonly used term. Legal blindness is defined as central visual acuity of 20/200 or less in the better eye with correcting lenses; or central visual acuity of more than 20/200 if there is a field defect in which the field has contracted to such an extent that the widest diameter of visual field represents an angular distance no greater than 20 degrees. It may be useful for legal or bureaucratic purposes, but as a description it is inadequate. In a very gross way, the person who is classified as legally blind can see no more than ten percent of what the person with normal sight can see.

Such a person will find it difficult, if not impossible, to read normal sized print. If his visual acuity is at the lower end of the range, he will not be able to travel, tell time, or do a hundred things without using special devices or receiving special training. Further, the limit on field vision in the descriptive term "legal blindness" sometimes contributes to misunderstanding. Although the visually impaired person may have quite good distance vision, his visual field is so restricted that he will have difficulty in performing tasks that normally require a wide field vision. He can read print, but he can see only a few words or symbols at a time. He then has to accommodate with increased head or eye movement for the restriction in his visual field. Anyone casually observing such a person might not know why he is classified as blind.

The picture is further complicated because the restriction may be central to the field or it may be peripheral; that is, the person may be able to see straight ahead but not to either side. On the other hand, he may have no central vision but can see objects to one side or the other. He may also have a condition known as "tunnel vision" or "pinhole vision," in which the effect is similar to that of trying to watch a ball game through a knothole in the fence. In all of these conditions the person retains some useful vision but is classified as legally blind.

The term *legal blindness* can be a useful indicator that a person is visually in a problem area. Anyone who has lost so much sight that he is even close to the standard is in trouble. However, one unfortunate aspect of the term is that when it is applied too rigidly, it establishes an arbitrary cutoff point. The person has lost enough sight to interfere with his ability to function at home, at work, or at play; he needs assistance in retraining or with information concerning special devices that will restore his functioning ability. He should not be denied this help simply because he is not quite legally blind. In the interest of accurate description, the term blindness should be reserved for those conditions in which loss of sight is complete or the remaining vision is so slight that it contributes little to the person's ability to function.

The term *severe visual impairment* should be used to describe those who retain large object perception or who can travel without a white cane or guide dog. This term would also apply to those who are not classified as legally blind. But, the specific term to be used is not nearly so important as the recognition that any severe or sudden loss of sight demands a physical, emotional, and social adjustment. Any drastic change in life circumstances, body functioning, or relationship to the environment requires that a person make some adaptation in order to cope with the change. This fact is not unique to severe or sudden visual impairment, but it is a relevant consideration for the person who loses his sight, as well as to those with whom he comes in contact.

The degree of sight remaining to the individual is, of course, relevant when considering his ability to function. If a person's visual acuity has been reduced beyond a certain point, he will simply not be able to read or do some other things that require sight. He might still be able to travel but he cannot do this safely without some identification such as a white cane or guide dog. If his field of vision is sufficiently restricted, he might be able to see objects at a distance, but he cannot drive safely. If he is completely blind, he will have to depend on his remaining senses for his ability to function, or depend on some sighted person to provide whatever help he needs. If he cannot read visually, he must learn to read braille or be read to by a sighted person.

STATISTICAL INFORMATION CONCERNING LEGAL BLINDNESS AND VISUAL IMPAIRMENT

Prevalence

The figures most often quoted concerning the prevalence of blindness or severe visual impairment are those provided by the National Society for the Prevention of Blindness. In a booklet titled Estimated Statistics on Blindness and Vision Problems the Society estimated that in the year 1978 there were 489,900 blind persons in the United States (employing the definition of legal blindness to describe the blind population). The estimate for the year 1980 is that there will be 519,200 blind persons in this country. The number of new cases for the year 1978 alone was expected to be 45,900. It should be noted, however, that these are not the actual data but are projections based on estimates by Dr. Ralph Hurlin in 1937, who indicated himself that the estimates are not satisfactory substitutes for factual measurements. It is, however, difficult to obtain hard data on such a large population.

Additional information concerning the prevalence of severe visual impairment comes from a survey conducted by the National Health Survey. According to this survey conducted during the period from July 1959 to June 1960, there were 988,000 persons with severe visual impairment in the United States. In this survey, the criterion for and the definition of severe visual impairment was the inability to read ordinary newsprint even with the aid of glasses. Such a loose definition without the control of relevant variables such as lighting undoubtedly results in overestimation of the problem. However, it still serves as an indicator of the magnitude of the problem.

AGE FACTORS IN VISUAL IMPAIRMENT

The estimates provided by the National Society for the Prevention of Blindness also give information concerning prevalence of visual impairment according to age. For the year 1962 it was estimated that there were 38,860 legally blind under the age of twenty. In the same year there were an estimated 54,040 between the ages of twenty and thirty-nine, and 117,890 between the ages of forty and sixty-four. Over the age of sixty-five there were an additional 188,510. The total for 1962 was 399,300.

It is readily apparent that there is a sharp increase in the prevalence of blindness beyond the age of forty. Thus, the onset of blindness or severe visual impairment compounds the problem for a person who is already at a disadvantage in the job market because of his age. For those who are beyond the normal age of retirement, the loss of sight adds a further complication in the aging process.

INADEQUACY AND SIGNIFICANCE OF THE DATA

The difficulty in attempting to extract some meaning from the available data is that they do not give an exact picture of the problem. It is for this reason difficult to evaluate the full extent of the needs or services required by this population.

Although the data leave much to be desired, they do at the very least give an indication of the magnitude of the problem. They suggest that the population of blind or visually impaired persons is much larger than might be supposed from the low profile of this group in the general population. They further suggest that the group is large enough to have a marked effect on the larger society. It is for this reason that greater consideration must be given not only to the physical needs of this group but also to the emotional needs of those who have lost their sight.

LOSS, DEPRIVATION, AND THE
EFFECTIVE USE OF REMAINING SIGHT

All persons who retain useful vision are not equal in their ability to use it effectively. One individual who retains only shadow perception seems to function quite well. He avoids objects while walking, or confidently reaches for something he wishes to pick up. Another individual with more vision gives the appearance of being helpless. He stumbles against objects, cannot find a door, or fumbles around when trying to pick up an object. He may barely be legally blind, but seems to be blinder than the person with minimal shadow perception. The difference between the two is the way in which they use their remaining sight. The one knows he must be approaching a door, because by the size and shape of the shadow it cannot be a window or piece of furniture. He looks competent because he does a good job of interpreting what he sees. The other person who appears to be less competent does not modify his behavior to use his remaining sight to its best advantage. Because he does not scan the area to either side of his field of vision, he misses objects he is looking for. He fumbles for his cup or gropes for a doorknob. As a result, he seems lost and clumsy. His remaining sight is not as useful, because he does not use it effectively.

In order to know how effectively a visually impaired person is using his remaining vision, it is important to know what this sight consists of. What part of the visual field is affected? Is the remaining sight clear, or is it blurred and distorted? How much is it affected by contrast or background? Some conditions or diseases give clues. *Retinitis pigmentosa*, for example, causes night blindness. No matter what the person can see in daylight, he is totally blind in the dark, or in dim light. If he passes from a well lighted room to a dimly lighted area, it will take a long time for his eyes to adjust to the change. The person may retain fairly good distance vision, but his *field of vision* is greatly restricted. *Retinal hemorrhages* may produce blurred vision so the person seems to be looking through a screen or fog. Shapes of objects are indistinct. In other cases, a hemorrhage blocks large areas of the field, leaving only small areas or patches of vision. In the case of *glaucoma*, the field also constricts so the person may eventually retain only *tunnel vision.* As a result, there are special problems of adaptation according to the condition. If a person sees only large blurred objects, he has a problem of interpretation: What is the object? How far away is it? If the person has a small clear area of useful sight, he knows what he sees, but does not know what may be just outside of this area. He must accommodate with appropriate head or eye movements.

In most cases, the adaptive solutions depend on whether or not the person is in familiar surroundings. In his own home, the person with blurred vision sees the object he knows to be a table, but may not be sure of his distance from it; so he uses a hand in a defensive technique to touch it as he approaches. In unfamiliar surroundings, he might not know what the object is, but might guess correctly. If, for example, he knows he is in an office, he can guess that the dark object is a desk. Also in unfamiliar surroundings, he walks toward the dark area he assumes to be a door and approaches it in such a way that he can reach for a door knob. By combining touch and good interpretation, he looks *competent.*

There are a number of reasons for this difference between individuals. Some persons do not *adapt* readily to change. They have fixed behavior patterns in which they persist, even though change would be more effective. An example of this is the person who clings to the speech patterns of childhood through high school and college even though better language would improve his ability to communicate. Others have emotional reasons for not making effective use of remaining vision. A self-conscious individual might feel that unusul head or eye movements or the use of special reading devices would attract unwanted attention. A person with a need to be dependent finds that when he fumbles for objects or bumps into things, he quickly gets the help he wants.

Depression is a strong reason for maintaining ineffectual behavior. The seriously depressed person feels that almost everything he does requires tremendous effort. He is too engrossed with his feelings of loss to concentrate on how he is using his remaining vision. He simply lets things happen and is indifferent to the consequences. Where emotional reasons are the basis for ineffective use of remaining sight, it is necessary to resolve the feelings before action toward changing the behavior will be effective. Whether through better interpretation, changes in behavior, or through the use of special aids, *every person should be helped* to make effective use of the sight he retains.

THE PROCESS OF LOSS

The way in which a person loses his sight varies according to the medical condition. One person may lose his sight suddenly, as the result of an accident or a retinal hemorrhage. Another person may lose his sight gradually over a period of years of steady deterioration. A third person may lose his sight within months because of untreated glaucoma. The condition may stabilize at some point following a drastic or sudden loss, or it may fluctuate from time to time between gradual losses and occasional but slight remission. Whatever the physical pattern may be, it will have its emotional effect on the person who is experiencing the loss.

CONGENITAL BLINDNESS

The effect of visual handicap is of course different for the person who is born blind or who loses his sight at a very early age. For him, the problem is one of normal growth and development within the limitation or deprivation that results from little or no sight. He does not have to make an adjustment to a new way of functioning after having learned to live and cope with his environment as a sighted person. The condition itself is normal for him. It is the way he perceives and has always perceived his environment. No change has taken place. However, if he is born with some sight and at a later time loses it, he must also make an adjustment to a more difficult way of functioning and will react emotionally to the new situation.

SECTION II

THE EMOTIONAL REACTION
TO THE
LOSS OF SIGHT

CHAPTER 3

REACTION TO LOSS

There is no "psychology of blindness" as a unique set of emotional responses to the loss of sight. The feelings that stem from severe visual loss are the same feelings that may be present in response to any event that constitutes a serious loss for anyone. If a close friend or family member dies, the survivor may experience shock, grief, or depression. If a person is unexpectedly fired from a job, it is possible that he will experience considerable devaluation. If through illness or danger the life of a child is threatened, the parents will almost certainly feel tremendous anxiety. The same application can be made to almost any emotion within the range of human experience.

The unique quality of any loss or physical disability does not lie in the feelings it generates, but in the special problems that result from it and in the meaning the loss has for the individual. The death of a close family member, first of all, is the loss of someone who is irreplaceable. If in addition he is the family breadwinner, his death has an immediate practical effect, since the family no longer has an income.

If the person loses a hand or an arm, he can no longer function as he did with both hands and arms. What he picks up and how he does so is affected by the loss. If he loses a foot or a leg, he cannot walk as he formerly did. In order to move about he must hobble or hop until he obtains an artificial limb. In either case his initial movements will be awkward. He will, to some extent, be dependent on others until he has acquired skill in using the prosthesis. In addition, the physical disability will have some meaning for him that will stimulate feelings in reaction to the loss. He will certainly experience frustration in his attempts to function. He may feel quite self-conscious because he looks and feels different. He will also feel that he is less of a person. Whatever the feelings may be, they are a consequence of what he has experienced and the way the loss affects his life.

19

When a person loses all or most of his sight, it is a serious and emotionally painful event. It will have an immediate effect on how he lives and what he does. It will also affect his feelings about himself and his relationship with others. In one way or another, it will affect almost every area of his life. A loss that so totally affects his life inevitably produces an emotional reaction. If he experiences the *loss*, he will certainly feel its effect. What he feels and how he reacts will be somewhat different from what another person feels and how he reacts. However, many of the feelings are shared by most persons who experience the loss of sight as well as by others who experience different but equally devastating losses.

The specific features of the *emotional reaction* as well as its intensity will be influenced by a number of internal and external factors. The individual will certainly be affected by the suddenness and severity of the loss. He will respond in terms of his unique personality characteristics. He will also be influenced by the way in which his family and friends react to his experience. In addition, he will be affected by what the community thinks and feels about blindness or visual impairment.

His first reaction will be based primarily on personality factors. That is, he will deal with the loss as he normally would deal with any personal crisis. In addition, the loss of sight will have some special meaning for him and this will be a determinant in the special emotional features that will be present in his reaction. As he begins to grapple with his feelings and the reality of his loss, the *family* will play an increasingly important role in how he feels about what is happening to him. They can cushion the impact of his experience if they are supportive in their response. If they are rejecting and critical, they will add to his feelings of aloneness. If, on the other hand, they are *overprotective*, they will add to his feelings of devaluation. The third factor that affects his continuing reaction to the loss of sight is the way in which members of the larger society react to his condition. If he loses his job because of his visual handicap, or if his friends avoid him, he will have to cope with an additional problem. He is then confronted with the fact that what has happened to him makes a difference to others. He may interpret the rejection as stemming directly from his visual impairment.

Thus, the visually impaired person finds that certain facts relating to a specific event have greatly affected his life situation. He has experienced a physical or organic change that has a direct bearing on his ability to deal with his physical environment. In addition, his social relationships are altered. The events are, or seem to be, beyond his control. Because of the effect they have on him and his feeling of helplessness in the face of these events, he reacts emotionally because he is a feeling being.

The feelings or emotions he experiences constitute reactions to a specific event . . . in the present case, the severe loss of sight. Their presence or absence varies from one individual to another. They may appear at different points in time following a drastic loss of sight. One person may display many of the responses described here while another person almost never displays them, but holds them in check while in the presence of others. Most persons who lose their sight will experience many of the reactions. As a reaction to an event that is as serious as the drastic loss of sight, they are entirely reasonable and understandable.

EMOTIONAL FACTORS ARE COMPLEXLY RELATED

Although I have isolated and analyzed the various factors that constitute the emotional reaction to the loss of sight as separate entities, I have done so only for the purpose of convenience and clarity. In fact, they do not function independently of each other. Where any of them are present in a particular individual, they are complexly related. The presence of one will affect the other emotional features that are present. It, in turn, is affected by still others. A specific reaction such as *depression* can be exacerbated by anxiety or frustration.

Furthermore, it is important to note that all of these factors are not present in every person who loses his sight. Often many of them are present in the same individual, but there is no way of predicting which will appear or which will be predominant at any given time. During the process of counseling, for example, it is possible to identify as separate entities some of the emotional features that attend the loss of sight. However, it is essential to be aware of the total interaction between these internal forces as well as the external forces that modify them.

CHAPTER 4

SHOCK AND REGRESSION

"... At first I thought the room was dark ... then I began to remember. The accident ... my boyfriend swerving to keep from hitting the dog ... we hit a tree. I remember being slammed against the windshield ... I wasn't wearing my seat belt. I wasn't knocked out, but it was all like a bad dream ... I couldn't see anything anymore ... Someone pulled me out of the car and put me on a stretcher ... Later they gave me a shot and said they would have to operate ... I reached up to my face and felt the bandages ... After a long time the doctor came in ... He told me my eyes were damaged. I was afraid to ask how bad ... I don't even remember the words he used, but it was like another shock ... like the accident all over again ... I felt as though he was talking to someone else ... It was still like a dream ... It wasn't happening to me. Even though the doctor never used the word, I think I knew I was going to be blind. But it was all so unreal. It was that way for three or four days. They gave me pills and I slept a lot. And whenever I'd wake up, it was a nightmare again because it wasn't me that was in that bed. It was all happening to someone else. A little at a time I knew it was me and I started thinking about what it would be like when they took the bandages off. And I began to believe when they did I'd still be able to see — at least a little. It's been over a month now and I still get the feeling once in a while that it's just a bad dream and I'll wake and everything will be alright."

SHOCK AS A RESPONSE TO LOSS

The phenomenon of shock is undoubtedly a protective mechanism. It is literally a blocking out of pain or sensation. Although it is well known as a response to physical injury, it occurs just as certainly as a response to emotional injury. The injury may be the loss that is felt when a close member of the family or a close friend *dies;* it may come in response to the loss of a job, or it may occur when some cherished hope is suddenly destroyed.

The severity of the shock experienced by a person is determined to some extent by the significance to him of what he has lost. One person can lose thousands of dollars and shrug it off as unimportant. Another person can lose one week's pay and feel as if he has just been dealt a severe blow. One person can be devastated by the death of a family member or the threat of divorce, while another person gives no apparent indication that he has been touched by either.

A second factor that determines the severity of shock may be the suddenness or unexpectedness of the event. A *death* that occurs suddenly can be a tremendous shock if the person who has died was apparently in good health. The shock might not be as great if he has been ill for a long time and the death was expected.

The person who experiences emotional shock will often describe the feeling as one of unreality. He sometimes refers to the nightmare quality of the experience. It is, in a sense, a frozen state in which he may feel detached from himself as a person. "I can't believe it's happening to me. It's as though I'm watching someone else." In this "frozen state" the individual has an opportunity to set aside what seems to be an unbearable reality. Cholden suggests that the shock period is a time for the person to mobilize his resources for the coming ordeal. He has time to assimilate the "real" facts in a gradual manner. He can delay the confrontation with reality until he feels he is able to cope with it. Shock, in this sense, is a defense mechanism that protects the individual against the possible disintegration of his personality. He has time to reorganize his thoughts and feelings. In the process, he integrates the event he has just experienced. The shock felt by a person suddenly losing a major portion of his sight is no less real because it is not the result of a physical blow or an accident. The loss affects what the person is and what he does. For this reason he will experience shock no matter what the medical cause of his loss.

As in all cases of emotional shock, the suddenness of the onset of blindness is a factor that determines the severity of the shock. The loss may be due to retinal homorrhage or it may be the result of an accident, but if the loss is sudden, the person has had no time to prepare for this eventuality and feels its full impact. If the loss had occurred more gradually, or in several stages, the individual might have had some forewarning and would have been able to prepare emotionally for the eventuality of further loss. Similarly, the degree of visual loss will affect the extent to which the individual feels the shock. If a person loses his sight completely as well as suddenly, he will experience greater shock than he will if the loss occurs in several stages over a period of time. Again, the mitigating factor is the opportunity to absorb the meaning of the event. In addition, the significance of the loss of sight to the individual will have a strong bearing on the severity of the shock he experiences. For most persons the loss of sight has psychological as well as practical significance. Where the psychological significance is great, the shock will be great. However, to the person for whom the loss is not as significant or to one who has a denial mechanism, the shock will not seem as great.

Whenever shock occurs, it provides an opportunity for disengagement from reality. The disengagement, however, is usually only temporary. Gradually, the feeling of shock diminishes, reality asserts itself, and the individual proceeds through the other emotions that accompany the loss of sight.

REGRESSION

The person who suddenly loses his sight often displays regressive behavior. In a manner reminiscent of childhood, he may eat with his fingers, spend an inordinate amount of time in bed, and at times cry easily and excessively. Often when frustrated in his wishes, he may indulge in a temper tantrum. He may refuse the responsibility of normal decision making, and may even expect to be dressed and have his clothes selected for him. Even shaving may appear to be so difficult that he will want to have a family member to perform the task for him.

The basis for such behavior is usually a need for reassurance.

It is a way of counteracting the feelings of devaluation that accompany serious loss of sight. What he may be saying by his behavior is, "When you give me the help I feel I need, you show me that you believe I am still a worthwhile person and you care about me. I am someone who deserves to be helped."

Regressive behavior certainly produces conflict for the family members who must deal with the needs or demands of the blind person. If they cater to the demands, they may feel they are reinforcing the behavior. They are afraid it will be maintained long beyond any reasonable period of time for adjustment. If they do not cater to it, they are left with a feeling of guilt or a nagging thought that they have not met the legitimate needs of the person who has lost his sight. Furthermore, if the behavior occurs in the presence of a third person such as a friend or acquaintance, they may feel they will be condemned for their heartless treatment of the "poor" blind person.

In fact, some regressive behavior is an unavoidable and normal consequence of the drastic, sudden loss of sight. It is difficult to use knife and fork when a lifetime of experience has always included vision to coordinate hand movements. Similarly, it is easy to become disoriented even in your own home when you have always depended on vision to orient yourself in relation to various objects. Furthermore, it is not unreasonable to cry over a loss as serious as that of sight.

The critical point for judging the reasonableness of regressive behavior is the length of time it persists and the person's willingness to attempt to change the behavior. The changes might not be great, but there should be gradual improvement. The improvement, of course, will be facilitated through psychotherapy or counseling. It would not be unreasonable to indulge the newly blinded person to some extent during the early stages of his adjustment. The person will then be assured of his worth as an individual. However, such reassurance should be accompanied with encouragement toward the ultimate goal of relative independence.

Making an evaluation of the person's condition requires considerable perception and sensitivity. It should properly be made by a professional knowledgeable in the problems of visual impairment.

CHAPTER 5

DEVALUATION AND SELF-CONSCIOUSNESS

The devaluation of self that occurs following major loss of sight must be considered in terms of the factors that contribute to a feeling of self-esteem. These factors originate in the values of society and are grounded in the developmental years of childhood. It is through such values as well as through the relationship with his parents that the individual builds an image of himself. He may not be able to verbalize what he feels, but his behavior will demonstrate what the feelings are. He lives, acts, or refrains from action on the basis of these feelings. As these change, his behavior will also change.

During early childhood, the individual is in an extremely dependent and helpless position. Almost every need must be met by another person. An adult, whether parent or surrogate, makes almost every decision for him. As the child grows, he becomes aware of himself and his relationship to others. His beginning struggles for autonomy are often frustrated because an adult decides that some bit of behavior of the child is not in his best interests or interferes with the adult's activity.

If the child wants approval, he must modify his behavior or delay gratification of his wishes. He must give up something he wants or wait to get it. He must conform to the wishes and whims of others. Because of his small size and relative help-lessness he must acquiesce when he would prefer to assert himself. He learns to cooperate in order to obtain the approval that is essential for a feeling of security. In time, he equates his feelings about himself — his self-esteem — with the approval of his parents.

If he continues to mature, he learns that productivity on his part elicits approval. He does small chores around the house and yard; he learns to read and write. He learns to take care of himself and is rewarded for achievement in his school work. His productive behavior is reinforced as he receives pay for doing useful work. Academic achievement has already become a means of maintaining or increasing self-esteem.

Then, such a person loses a major portion of his sight and suddenly the factors that contributed to his self-esteem become the measure of his inferior status. The standard is now a way of demonstrating his inadequacy as a contributing member of society. He can no longer read and write. As a father and husband it may be difficult, if not impossible to provide for his family. A wife and mother initially cannot shop or do household tasks without assistance. Thus, the person is prevented from contributing in the expected manner and has lost the basis for receiving the approval he needs.

In our culture most people are expected to work and earn their living. However, there are few ways of earning a living that are not directly affected when a person loses a major portion of his sight. A bus or truck driver would lose his job immediately. An engineer would not be able to read blueprints. A doctor or a nurse could not treat patients without the ability to read charts and medication labels. Thus, the immediate consequence of the loss of sight is loss of income.

For many people the only alternative is to apply for welfare. This in itself can be, and in most cases is, a devaluing experience. A person who once earned a good living and spent his income as he wished now must ask for assistance. He must live on a subsistence income and account to a stranger for his everyday needs. Such a person has absorbed cultural attitudes toward welfare. He has had at least minimal acquaintance with such attitudes as, "Any worthwhile person works for a living," or "Get goldbrickers off the welfare rolls." It is no consolation that such criticism usually excludes blind persons. The fact that blind persons are excused from the expectations is demonstrable proof that they are dependent and helpless. They should be cared for because, in some way, they are inferior. Society sets aside many normal expectations because blind people are thought incapable of meeting normal standards.

Thus, the necessity of accepting welfare adds to other factors that lead to lowered self-esteem.

AUTONOMY

The person who can see has the option of initiating social contacts whenever he chooses to do so. He can walk over and talk with acquaintances when he sees them in a restaurant, at the club, or on the street. At a social gathering he can walk over and talk with another person even if the other person would prefer to avoid him because he is a bore. Because of this freedom, he can at least maintain the illusion that he has friends.

Without sight, a person is more completely dependent on the interest and willingness of others to make the contacts. He cannot scan the faces in a club or restaurant to find a familiar one. At a party, he must wait for people to approach him, because he is not familiar enough with his surroundings to walk about freely. Acquaintances will often fail to invite him, either because they are uncomfortable in his presence, or because they do not know what to do with him.

As his circle of acquaintances constricts and he receives fewer and fewer invitations, he may conclude that he is not the kind of a person other people wish to see. It is even more likely that he will assume his blindness is the reason people avoid him. This assumption is devastating because it is the one thing he cannot change. In either case, because he has fewer contacts with other people than formerly, he feels like less of a person.

AGE FACTORS IN DEVALUATION

I am frequently asked, "What is the worst age at which to lose your sight?" Sometimes the young client will take the approach that at least he is young enough to choose a career that is feasible for one with limited vision. Or he may feel that he still has the energy and strength to cope with his difficulties. The person in his middle years may feel that he already has a family to help and also has the necessary experience to live with his problem. He may feel that his position is more advantageous than that of an elderly person because of the future that is still possible for him. The elderly person may feel that he has had many good years of visual experience. He has pleasant memories of things he has done and things he has seen. He thinks it must be terrible for the person who loses his sight while still young and who has "all those years of being blind ahead of him." Or he thinks he is lucky that he does not have the responsibility of raising a family after losing his sight.

Conversely, many people in each of these groups may concentrate on the special problems each of them has at his particular age. A young person wishes he could have kept his sight long enough to become established in a career and start a family. The middle-aged peson feels burdened by the responsibility of raising a family or training for a new occupation without sight. The elderly person wishes he could have kept his sight for the few remaining years. He might comment that he could have handled his problems better when he was younger. "It's hard to teach an old dog new tricks." In fact, each age has its special problems. All of the comments expressed are, in a way, correct, and in a way, they are not correct. The painfulness of the experience is a function of what the person is able to feel, the practical consequences of the loss, and what the loss means to him personally. The devaluation that the individual feels is not imaginary. It is real because the loss of sight does not improve his status or circumstances. It does not, in itself, make him a stronger or better person. Clearly, it makes him physically less than he was prior to the loss of sight. In time, he may adjust to the loss or compensate for it, but the devaluation is based on emotional, physical, and social reality.

THE ADOLESCENT

The adolescent is chronologically very close to the dependent period of childhood. He has now reached the time for attempting to establish autonomy by gradually separating himself from the control of his parents. He is in the process of trying to find himself as a person. If at this critical period he loses his sight, he is again forced into the dependent role of the child. In his struggle to retain the independence and freedom he has barely tasted, he may become rebellious or perverse simply as a reaction to the distasteful dependent role.

The dominant reference group for the adolescent is his peer

group. He looks to the group, or to certain members of it, for approval. However, he also competes for status and position within the group. Some forms of behavior among teenage boys are designed to impress girls and get their attention. Dating is often a means to establish status — as when a boy is able to date a particularly popular girl. Physical activity is another means of competing among teenage males. By running, jumping, and swimming they demonstrate physical prowess, and use their accomplishments as a way of comparing themselves with others in the group. They not only drive cars, but do so in ways to prove their ability and fearlessness.

When such a boy loses his sight, he is no longer able to compete on the same level. At best, he is at a disadvantage in competing with sighted friends. Even with some residual vision, he is forced to compete on an unequal level. If he has difficulty seeing where he is going, he cannot run, jump, or swim with the same ease. He is more limited in his ability to function. At worst, if he has lost his sight completely, he cannot even enter into competition except in some very limited areas. Even apart from the feelings that intefere with his ability to date, he does not have the opportunity or the means to date easily, as other teenage boys do. Since he is unable to drive, he does not have this means of pitting himself against the abilities of others. Nor does he have the stories or experience to relate to his friends. He suddenly finds himself on the periphery of activity.

To some extent, the adolescent girl finds herself in the same predicament when she loses her sight. Boys may hesitate to ask her for a date because they are uncomfortable and do not know how to interact with a blind or visually handicapped girl. If she does not date regularly, she has less to discuss with other girls. In addition, she feels she is less attractive. She may be just as attractive as other girls, but how can she know this?

Of course, many persons feel inferior in looks or ability regardless of the reality of their condition. But the problem is more critical for the teenage girl who has not yet established a good self-image. As in the case of adolescent boys, the visually impaired teenage girl is in an inferior position in any situation in which she might compete with her friends. If she has sight, she can compare her physical appearance and the things she does with those of others. Without sight, she loses this opportunity for comparison. She must depend on the judgment of others for self-evaluation. This dependence places her in a difficult position. The other person's judgment may be valid, but how does she know what experience the other person has for making the judgment? She knows what her own experience has been, but it is no longer available to her without sight. All the cues for controlling the environment that are available to most people are no longer available to her.

THE MIDDLE YEARS

The middle years have their own special problems. As an adult, the individual has already passed through the turmoil of adolescence. Usually, he has established an identity and achieved an independent status. His personality traits are defined and he has gained some confidence in his own abilities. In most cases, he has assumed the responsibility of marriage and a family. In all likelihood, he has begun a career or has established himself in a job or occupation. A woman in this same age range has essentially achieved the same goals. She may have a career; she may be a wife. If she is a mother, her children may be young or almost grown. She has a concept of herself in her various roles. The feeling that these various men and women have about their identity is based not only on what they feel they are, but also on their abilities and accomplishments. Following the loss of sight, all this changes. Their life situation becomes fluid or unstable. They can no longer do the things they have always done. Their confidence in themselves and their future is shaken. The future is uncertain because in most cases their work — and ultimately their goals — are in jeopardy. Their confidence dissolves as their independence is undermined and their status in the community is threatened. Under the circumstances, it is then no wonder that they think less of themselves as individuals than they did formerly. They find it difficult to meet the crisis that has been presented by the severe loss of sight, and as a result, their self-esteem is lowered.

THE ELDERLY

The elderly person also has his special set of problems. He already feels he is being "phased out." He is no longer in the mainstream of activity. Physically and mentally he knows that he is not as capable as he once was. Health and strength are failing. He is susceptible to the illnesses that attend the aging process. He is all too aware of his diminished resources and worth to the community. In our society, he is left with little to do after he retires. He may occasionally visit his children or grandchildren, but often they live separate, active lives. They are busy; he has time to spare. If the wife or husband dies, he may feel that time is running out for him. As he loses friends, his circle of activity shrinks. Because of his age, he is already experiencing many of the elements that are the foundation of devaluation.

If, at this point in the process, he experiences the loss of all or most of his sight, or is even threatened with such loss, it is as though he has received a double blow. Not only has he been literally retired, but he finds that the loss of sight threatens to take away his remaining independence. As a blind or visually impaired elderly person, he feels even less worthwhile than he did simply as an elderly person. He cannot even freely attend or participate in many of the activities reserved for his group. He either feels that he is a burden on the family, or he feels that he is alone because no one really cares about him. He attributes this situation to his loss of sight — and his self-esteem suffers.

CHAPTER 6

REACTIVE DEPRESSION, SUICIDE AND LOSS OF SIGHT

The depressed person often presents a general demeanor of sadness. His speech and actions are slow and deliberate as though requiring great effort. He cries, and the crying is often precipitated by seemingly insignificant comments from a friend or family member. Furthermore, he may find it difficult to sleep, or alternatively, may be inordinately sleepy much of the time. The comments he makes reflect a pessimistic attitude concerning almost every event or happening. He presents many complaints, such as his restricted activity or a lack of enjoyment in his relationships. His interests are narrowed and often his sex drive is diminished. Ordinary tasks become difficult, if not impossible, to perform. Unable to believe that there is any basis for hope, he perseverates on what he has lost.

The depressed mood may last for long periods of time, or it may occur for shorter but more frequent periods. It may last for only a few hours or days after the onset of blindness, or be delayed for a long period and then be precipitated by some apparently unconnected incident. The underlying cause is the loss of sight, but the connection between this and the precipitating event is not readily apparent. For example, a friend fails to keep an appointment, which seems to depress the visually impaired person, when in fact he is really depressed over the loss of his independence. In other cases, the precipitating event is directly related to the loss of sight. The person becomes depressed because his blindness prevents him from enjoying some visual experience.

The intensity of the depression is not necessarily evident in a superficial interview. The person often has a desire to hide what he is feeling because he is ashamed of it. He looks on the depression as a weakness or as an abnormal reaction to his loss, thinking, "Other people wouldn't feel this way." Such a person may attempt to hide his reaction except when he is alone, or when he is involved in counseling or psychotherapy. He may hide his depression even from close members of his family because he does not wish to burden them.

Others who may not actually be as severely depressed are more free to express their feelings. They cry readily and tell what they feel to anyone who is willing to listen. They display this behavior because they are less inhibited or because they want the sympathy of friends and family. Undoubtedly the motivation for this easy expression of depression is usually more complicated than this.

In the case of more severe depression the individual becomes more withdrawn — closed in — and is less concerned with the reactions of those around him. He feels extreme emotional pain and is absorbed with the intensity of the experience.

POINT OF ONSET

The point at which depression appears depends, to some extent, on the degree of loss and what this means to the individual. If the person experiences the full impact, as in the case of sudden and total loss, then depression usually follows quickly. If, however, sufficient sight remains to minimize the real effect of blindness, the person does not have to face the full meaning of his condition, and he might not have any "real" reason for becoming depressed. The condition as yet, has no meaning for him. He may then give the appearance of being well-adjusted. As long as he retains sufficient sight, he can maintain the fiction of normality. He denies the reality of his visual loss and convinces himself that he is functioning quite well with his remaining vision. But if his sight deteriorates further, he is forced to deal with the limitations of his condition. In other words, the reactive depression results only if the degree of visual loss is sufficient to force the individual to deal with the frustration of his loss.

On the other hand, even persons with considerable remaining vision may react with deep depression to the loss of sight. They may compare their present degree of vision with what they had formerly. What they have now is not as important as what they have already lost. Thus, the point of emotional impact is in part the product of the actual loss and in part the psychological meaning of the loss to the individual.

MOURNING

Mourning, in most cases, is an integral part of the depressive reaction following the loss of sight. Other writers have described the phenomenon.[1,5] They usually discuss the reaction as one of dying to an old way of life and being born again to a new one. Although some writers might question the validity of such a phenomenon, many clients describe their feelings in terms that clearly indicate that they are experiencing mourning. One such client stated, "I feel just the way I did when my mother died." Frequently I have heard other clients verbalize their feelings with comments such as, "I feel as though this is the end of my life." Such unsolicited comments are a clear indication of the ongoing mourning process.

Mourning is in itself a complicated process. It represents a feeling of loss for the individual and is expressed as a feeling of grief or sadness. It also includes feelings of guilt over what the person believes to have been unworthy thoughts or actions. In addition, the grief that the person feels is evidence that what he lost was worthwhile or precious.

Mourning usually follows the loss of an object. Most persons associate the presence of mourning with the death of a close friend or relative. However, the loss of a material object or a part of the body can also precipitate a mourning reaction. The important features of a relationship do not have to be on a conscious level. Many of the reasons for the attachment may have symbolic or unconscious significance. Similarly, every part of the body is invested with special meaning. The sum of all of these is the "I" that is my body and my mind. Each part makes its special contribution to the concept of "self." "If I lose any part of my body I am no longer exactly what I was prior to the loss. I cannot function precisely as I used to."

It is usually accepted as natural to grieve when a close friend or family member dies. It is just as natural to grieve over the loss of some body part. In addition to whatever special meaning the body part had for the person, the loss usually involves a drastic change in his ability to function. His habitual pattern of activity is disrupted and this change in itself can be very disturbing.

A further cause for grief at the death of a friend or family member can be a reminder to the individual that he too is mortal. Similarly, the loss of an important sense or part of his body is an immediate reminder of this fact. If he loses a leg or an arm, he knows that part of him has died. If he loses his sight, it has the same significance. In addition, he has lost an important means of contact with his environment and he knows that some day he will lose contact with everything that is familiar.

Such thoughts are not easily accessible to consciousness. But to the extent to which they are, the person will anticipate his death. In this sense, as he mourns the loss of his sight, he mourns for himself. In his grief, he combines his feelings for what he has already lost with his feelings for what he will eventually lose. The mechanism is comparable to what one feels when a close person has an incurable disease. It is an anticipatory grief, but it is just as real as the grief he feels when the person actually dies. The anticipatory mechanism is also present in the depressive reaction that occurs when a person is in the process of losing his sight. He grieves over the sight he has already lost as well as over his eventual and total loss of sight.

The person who has lost something must come to terms with the loss and must learn to cope with the reality of its consequences. Thus, in the process of mourning he must give up what he has known and begin to live in a new way. The person who grieves is in this process of transition. Gradually, the emphasis shifts from what is behind to what is ahead. In the process, he moves into a new state of being. In this sense the mourning process is a normal and healthy reaction to a severe loss.

PUNISHMENT AS A BASIS FOR REACTIVE DEPRESSION

Many persons verbalize the belief that the loss of sight represents a punishment. God or an unkind fate is punishing them for unworthy acts or thoughts. Sometimes they can identify a specific act or thought for which they are being punished. However, in most cases their reason for the punishment is some vague or unidentified behavior. These persons are generally afflicted with an underlying feeling of guilt, and blindness becomes the focus and the justification for their feelings. It is the punishment for their unworthiness and the proof of their misdeeds.

Occasionally the loss of sight becomes an adequate punishment for unworthiness. The onset of blindness then relieves the need for self-castigation. When this occurs, the person is, in a sense, released from his bondage of guilt and can live and function in a productive manner. He no longer needs to do things, such as losing a job — a form of self-punishment.

This mechanism will operate only if blindness is an adequate punishment for unconscious guilt. This is demonstrated in the case of depressed individuals blind from self-inflicted gunshot wounds, who continue to live in a state of self-castigation. They demonstrate chronic depression centering around the feeling or belief that they are unworthy individuals. Their depression stems from unconscious guilt, and the blindness resulting from a self-inflicted gunshot wound does nothing to relieve this burden of guilt.

DEVALUATION AS A BASIS FOR DEPRESSION

Depression may also result from the devaluing effects that often attend the loss of sight. Such feelings are understandable since the person is no longer able to function as he once did. Now he is unable to do the things he used to do that formerly made him feel worthwhile — the things on which he built his image as a useful, independent person.

PROGNOSIS

Reactive depression is quite amenable to treatment. If the pessimistic attitude is dominant, the person can be helped to restructure his thinking concerning blindness or severe visual impairment. He may have to resign himself to permanent visual impairment when this is indicated by the medical prognosis. However, he need not resign himself to a permanent state of helplessness or dependency. The therapist can encourage him through a realistic appraisal of his potential. In turn, this understanding can be supported as the visually impaired person relearns old skills or through training, acquires new ones. As he discovers that he can again become a competent and useful person, the depressive mood will gradually lift and he will again resemble the person he was prior to the loss of sight.

SUICIDE AND LOSS OF SIGHT

Suicidal thoughts are common in persons who have experienced a serious loss of sight. Some individuals are quite frank in admitting that they have such thoughts, while others only allude to them as they discuss their difficulties. Still other persons express suicidal thoughts in the form of death wishes. They state that they want something to happen to them. They have the wish to "end it all" but do not want to commit the act themselves; they want some other agent to perform the act for them. "Sometimes I wish a car would run over me and it would be all over," or "I'm going on a trip and I wish the plane would crash."

In some cases, the person will speak quite bluntly about his suicidal intentions. One man who was in the process of losing his sight stated quite simply and coolly, "If I lose any more of my sight, I'm going to kill myself. I won't live that way." He had a poor relationship with his wife on whom he would have to be dependent. The knowledge of this problem, in addition to the way in which he delivered the statement, made me feel quite certain that at this point in his life he meant what he said.

Others not only make the threat, but actually plan how they will kill themselves. One young man with a wife and two children described his plans for suicide: "When I first started losing my sight, I thought about driving my car over the edge of a cliff. I waited too long for that and now I can't do it because I can't drive anymore. What I've been thinking is that I'll go to the beach with the family, swim out a ways and let myself drown . . ."

During the next few sessions, we discussed his feelings regarding the loss of sight and how they related to his wish to commit suicide. We also discussed his relationship with his family and how it would affect them to see him drowning while they stood by helplessly. As he talked, he came to the conclusion that he did not want to hurt the children this way. In time, he also became aware of his worth to the family in spite of the certainty that he would eventually be totally blind.

With all such persons the suicidal thoughts are obviously on a conscious level. There is no doubt about the wish or the intent of the speaker. Others, however, may have death wishes but they are suppressed through the mechanism of denial. In addition, they may be projected on other family members. One client, a middle aged woman, stated that she did not mind flying. Almost immediately she began talking about one of her sons who had to go on many business trips and usually flew by commercial airliner. Whenever she knew he was on a trip, she constantly listened to the news because she expected to hear that a plane had crashed. She made these comments while discussing the difficulty and anxiety she was experiencing because of her loss of sight.

Suicidal thoughts and death wishes are usually more evident during the depressive phase following visual loss. As the mood of the individual lifts, however, there is less emphasis on thoughts of dying or the wish to end it all. Gradually, the focus changes from the morbid and hopeless here and now to the hope or goal of a satisfying life even with impaired vision.

FACTORS CONTRIBUTING TO SUICIDAL THOUGHTS

A number of factors such as anxiety, hostility, and dread of abandonment contribute to suicidal thoughts. Anxiety may stem from the person's doubt that he can cope with further loss of sight. The unknown frightens him and he wishes only to escape from the coming ordeal. He wishes he were already totally blind because he cannot deal with the anxiety of waiting, or he may wish to relieve the anxiety by escaping into death. Insofar as the loss of sight is a symbolic death, the reaction is comparable to that of the soldier who is so afraid of dying that he charges into the death he fears. In the case of the visually impaired person, the thought of death may seem, for a time, preferable to the difficulty of coping with further loss of sight.

There is usually some element of hostility or aggression in any suicidal wish or attempt. One elderly man was extremely depressed over the continuing deterioration of his sight. His wife became more and more controlling as his sight diminished. Eventually she made all the decisions concerning the places they went and the people they visited. She often refused to take him places he wished to go. She frequently thwarted his attempts to become independent. He was unable to sever the relationship because, in reality, he was very dependent on her. Several times during the course of counseling he became so angry at his wife that he threatened to commit suicide. The threat was both a way of escape and the ultimate weapon of his anger. Eventually, he resolved the feelings as he became aware that a realistic solution was possible through training and relative independence.

When dread of abandonment is the basis for suicidal thoughts or actions, the individual often gives away his feelings. He either tells the family what he intends to do or makes a tentative effort to commit suicide. In this roundabout way the person tells his family how he feels. One woman, a widow in her middle forties, is a case in point. She had two children in their middle and late teens. She was so disturbed by the fear that they would soon leave her that she attempted to commit suicide by running across a busy street against a red light. However, before running out of the house, she became hysterical and told her son what she intended to do. He ran after her and forcibly stopped her before she reached the street. In her hysterical state she expressed her feelings to her children. They had not been aware of her feelings and were shocked by her behavior and her words. Because of what she told them, she and her children were able to achieve better understanding of her fears and their mutual needs.

PREVENTION OF SUICIDE

When any person expresses suicidal thoughts or wishes, he should be taken quite seriously. Even an allusion to suicidal wishes should be carefully explored to determine the full extent of the person's intentions. Unfortunately, talk of suicide often arouses anxiety in the listener and he tends to avoid the subject with a reassuring, "Oh, you don't mean that," or some equally ineffective remark. Such an approach can be of no help to the person who has lost or is losing his sight and because of his distress may be considering taking an action as drastic as suicide.

The specific techniques for dealing with a potentially suicidal person are treated adequately in the literature.[8] If the situation seems critical, it is imperative to get help from some community service organization, such as the Los Angeles Suicide Prevention Center. In any case, the individual needs professional counseling to help him understand the basis for his feelings and to put him in touch with more constructive alternatives to his problems.

CHAPTER 7

ANXIETY

EXTERNAL DANGER

Two critical factors in the reaction to any serious loss of sight are the actual helplessness experienced by the person, and the expectation of helplessness if he should lose his remaining sight. In either case, the person does not believe he will be able to mobilize the resources he needs to function in a potentially dangerous situation. The danger may be real or it may be imagined, but the expectation of danger causes him to think about his helplessness. He is certain he will not be able to cope.

The person who has lived all his life with normal senses has learned to use them to control his environment and to move himself in relation to it. His ability to do so affects his well being, freedom, and survival. When he makes a mistake, he feels pain and discomfort. His "set" or attention has been directed toward self-protection. When he relaxes this attention, he is reminded that certain aspects of his environment can be dangerous or harmful. The anticipation he experiences because of this knowledge is anxiety.

Mild anxiety can facilitate a person's ability to function. The person who expects danger is more aware of threatening aspects of the environment. In fact, some concern for danger in the surroundings is essential for survival. When the individual feels anxiety, he watches for things that can harm him. If he wishes to jaywalk across a busy street, he may do so without anxiety if he is sufficiently nimble. He can even reduce whatever anxiety he feels if he notices a traffic signal down the street and is willing to walk a block out of his way. If he does not have the physical agility, his anxiety will certainly argue in favor of the longer route. In either case, he has made a choice after visually evaluating the situation. Since he cannot control the actions of motorists, he moves himself in relation to them in a manner designed to minimize danger and consequently anxiety.

In the same situation, the most obvious limitation for the visually impaired person is his inability to evaluate the situation and make a judgment regarding his actions. He hears the noise of traffic and possibly notices blurred objects rushing past him. If he is on an unfamiliar street, he may be uncertain about the location of a traffic light, which may be a block in either direction. Finding a suitable crossing place is, therefore, more difficult for him than it is for a person with sight. His anxiety level plus prudence — a function of anxiety — would probably not permit him to cross without a traffic light. He might assume that motorists seeing his white cane would stop. However, some might not notice the cane until too late. Furthermore, there is the possibility that some motorists do not know the meaning of the white cane. These are critical considerations if he is about to commit himself to the judgment of others, and without sight, he cannot compensate for what they might lack. The resulting anxiety would undoubtedly determine his actions in favor of seeking a safe crossing point.

On the other hand, if the anxiety is too great, it will interfere with his ability to function well while traveling. It might even prevent him from making the attempt to travel, in spite of the fact that he retains minimal vision or has received travel training.

GENERALIZED ANXIETY

Occasionally I have worked with clients who experienced a generalized anxiety response following the loss of sight. Because of their anxiety, they did not even attempt to travel. They refused to cook a meal because they were afraid they might burn themselves. They avoided attending social functions as much as possible. Some of these people were able to find their way around their own home, but when alone felt terribly anxious.

The age of the client did not seem to be a factor. Some of the clients who described this anxiety reaction were elderly, while others were young adults. One such case was that of a seventy five year old woman who was living with a married daughter. She would go everywhere with her daughter, even when it was inconvenient. She could not remain at home alone for more than a half hour without becoming exceedingly nervous. Another case was that of a young man who had lost his sight completely as the result of an accident. He stated that when-ever he was at home alone, he would get out his father's revolver because he was afraid someone might break into the house and he would be defenseless.

The underlying basis for the anxiety was complex in both cases. However, both clients talked much about their feelings of helplessness. They both felt the environment was dangerous and they were vulnerable to attack.

SITUATIONAL ANXIETY

Anxiety may result when a visually impaired person is in one specific situation or when he is forced to perform a specific task. He may feel quite comfortable or relaxed in familiar sur-roundings such as his home, but if he is forced to go out on a mobility lesson, he expeiences the sensation of butterflies in his stomach. His anxiety is reduced as he gains some compe-tence in traveling, but if he progresses to a new phase of his mobility training, he again feels anxious.

Case History — Stanley

Stanley, who had lost his sight as the result of glaucoma, was forty two years old at the time he came to the agency. He was married and had two teenage children. He discovered he was losing his sight when he had an accident while driving a truck. Prior to his loss, he was already aware of the meaning of blindness because his mother had been totally blind for several years as the re-sult of glaucoma.

At the time he began mobility training he still

retained approximately three percent of his sight, but with a considerably restricted field of vision. With this degree of vision he could see large objects although he could no longer identify the color of traffic lights.

As part of his mobility training he was required to work blindfolded with a white cane. He found this to be a very trying experience.

Interview with Stanley

(P stands for psychologist. C stands for client.)

P: How are you getting along in mobility?

C: I just got back from a lesson. It was — some lesson.

P: What happened?

C: I had to travel under a blindfold. I did it. But — I was scared as hell!

P: Was the instructor with you?

C: Yes, he was right behind me. But it wasn't that. I knew he wouldn't let me get hurt.

P: Do you have any idea why you were so frightened?

C: Yes...It made me realize what it would be like if I lose my sight completely.

P: And what would it be like?

C: It made me feel completely helpless. I didn't know what was happening around me.

P: But you were able to travel, even with a blindfold, weren't you?

C: Yeah, I guess that's true. I was scared, but I made it.

P: So you weren't completely helpless. Were you?

The mobility instructor later commented that
he had not been aware of the client's anxiety. On
this lesson, the client did not talk to the instruc-
tor about his feelings, and his movements were
sufficiently controlled to disguise them.

SOCIAL SITUATIONS

For the visually impaired person social situations may not
have the element of actual physical danger. However, in their
own way, they can be just as threatening for the person who
cannot see well enough to function independently. The threat
in these situations usually centers around the possibility of
embarrassment. The basis for the anxiety is the possibility of
social disapproval. The visually impaired person might expect
that others could be critical of the way he dresses, the quality of
his manners, or of something he might do that would draw
attention to his condition. He would probably be self-critical
because he is unsure of his ability to cope with whatever situation arises. He would, above all, dread the possibility that someone might ask questions that he is not ready to answer.

The difficulty for the newly blinded or visually impaired person is that he knows he cannot anticipate every eventuality,
especially if he is in a strange house. He cannot move about
freely because he might bump into another guest. If the group
is large and noisy, he will not be able to find someone he wishes
to speak to. If he wishes to go to the bathroom, he must ask
someone to show him the way. Any of these possibilities will
draw attention to him, and the possibility stimulates anxiety.

ANXIETY AND WORK

The person who is in the process of losing his sight may feel
considerable anxiety concerning the possibility that he will not
be able to perform on the job. Many employers hold negative
attitudes toward visually impaired persons, and he is aware of
this. He feels real anxiety because his financial independence
hinges on his ability to keep his job. I have known of some cases
in which people were able to function for several months on a
job in spite of a serious loss of sight. They were, however, in a
constant state of anxiety because a supervisor or superior

might learn of their visual condition. Unfortunately, in some of these cases, their fears were confirmed when they were terminated from employment after the employer learned of their disability. The anxiety the person felt at the possibility of losing his job was then replaced by the more basic anxiety regarding the means of supporting his family.

INSUFFICIENT CUES

With little or no sight, a person is forced to function with a considerable reduction in the amount of normally available information about the environment. In most situations sight is the predominant sense. With it, a person not only can gather information from a greater distance than he can with any other sense, but he can make finer discriminations than with either touch or hearing. Any feature of the environment that does not emit sound is available at a distance only through the medium of sight. The blind person can be standing relatively close to a large object without being aware of its presence. He can never be sure that activity is not taking place simply because he hears nothing. All he can know for certain is that no noise-emitting activity is taking place. This in itself can be the basis for the onset of anxiety, particularly if he is in unfamiliar surroundings. He strains to hear and wonders what is taking place, or what objects are around him.

Sight is an active sense. The person with normal sight can, at will, explore his surroundings and he can do this at close range or at some distance. Furthermore, he can do this without moving from his position. The important consideration is that the individual can initiate visual activity and this helps him to believe he can control his environment. He can defend himself, if necessary, against danger. The only exceptions are situations in which the sighted person is in almost darkness or in which, for other reasons, visibility is obscured.

Hearing is a passive sense. If a sound is not emitted or reflected by an object, the visually impaired person is unaware of its proximity. He is entirely dependent on the sound cues that the environment produces. He must listen, and if at the moment he is listening, there is no sound, he must depend on his sense of touch. The exception is in the case of close proximity to a large object such as a wall. It is possible to reflect sounds from it by whistling or snapping fingers.

Touch, like sight, is an active sense. The visually impaired person does not need to wait for information to be produced for him in order to learn something about the environment. The value of this sense, however, is limited because it is useful only at a close range. In addition, it is not possible to make the fine discriminations that can be made with sight. Furthermore, touch is inadequate when the desired information concerns a rapidly moving object. Thus, the visually impaired person is left without sight, the most useful sense, and is dependent on lesser senses — touch and hearing. They are useful but extremely limited when compared with sight. In many situations they do not provide sufficient information to prevent or allay anxiety.

This is not to say that a sighted person never experiences anxiety. Nor is it to say that a blind person cannot function without — or at least with minimal — anxiety. However, the great reduction in available information for a visually impaired person is a significant factor when considering the anxiety he experiences as he attempts to function actively within his environment.

DISTORTION OF CUES

The susceptibility of auditory cues to distortion is especially critical when the sense of hearing is the major source of information about the environment. If a jet plane roars overhead just as a visually impaired person is attempting to cross a street, all crucial traffic sounds are masked. The same thing happens if construction crews are working on the street with jack hammers or other noisy equipment just as he approaches an intersection. He cannot hear the normal flow of traffic which gives him the cue that the traffic light has changed. A motorist may be turning in front of him without his knowledge. Because he is left without the sounds that provide the cue of direction, he cannot be sure that he is not veering slightly from his intended course. If the sound is loud enough, he literally has no way of knowing what is happening and may be immobilized by caution or anxiety until the noise subsides.

The background noise may completely block out auditory

stimuli. However, it may be just sufficiently loud to distort them
or to make them ambiguous to the hearer. If, just as he starts to
cross a street, someone calls out but the words are not clear, he
may find himself in conflict. The person may be calling to him
because he is about to get into some danger or offering to help
him cross the street. On the other hand, the person may not be
addressing him at all. The situation, because it suggests some
possibility of danger, stimulates anxiety. If the anxiety is great
enough, he may not even attempt to cross the street until he receives help. He may even take the wrong action because of his
anxiety.

A similar situation can stimulate anxiety even in the relative
security of the home. The blind person who attempts to cook a
meal depends to some extent on his hearing to prevent injury
around a hot stove. If an exhaust fan is sufficiently loud, he may
have difficulty hearng the sound of something boiling or frying.
When he reaches for a pot or pan, he uses sound as well as heat
to orient himself to it, and to judge his distance from it. If he
misjudges the distance he may receive a slight burn. It requires
only an occasional contact with a hot object to perpetuate a
state of anxiety whenever the blind person must cook. The
anxiety may be rather mild but it can interfere with effective
functioning in a particular situation. Anxiety is most likely to be
present in the early stages of adjustment, while the person is
acquiring the skill or competence to perform well in this task.
The person with a severe visual impairment has few options in
such a situation. He can turn off the fan each time he must re-
move something from the stove. This, however, is not as easy to
do if the auditory interference is the noise of young children
screaming through the kitchen. He can also ask for help or ask
someone else to cook for him. The only other possibility is gradually to develop skill in the technique of cooking without sight
and to depend on other senses and aids to prevent injury.

A similar problem can occur when the blind person is attempting to find his way through the house while a vacuum
cleaner is in operation. The noise blocks out cues he may require to find his way around without bumping into doors or
wall corners. The sound he needs to hear may be that of a
loudly ticking clock that tells him the direction to a doorway; or
it may be the radio playing that gives him his orientation. The
anxiety that results from the blocking of such cues may cause

the person to become more tense. This will further decrease his ability to orient himself.

The presence of such anxiety may seem to be irrelevant as long as the person is attempting to function or to acquire the skills he needs for good adaptation. However, the anxiety a person feels is often a factor in the progress he makes, or in the resistance he demonstrates at the suggestion of acquiring a new skill. If he is attempting to function under the pressure of strong anxiety, it is doubtful that he will progress as quickly as he would without such anxiety. He is also more likely to make many mistakes in his performance.

ANXIETY AND FURTHER LOSS

Many persons who have lost a drastic amount of sight experience considerable anxiety when they consider the possibility that their sight may deteriorate further. The reaction is entirely understandable since they have lost so much. Once a serious loss has occurred, it is only too easy to believe that the same thing can happen again.

This is particularly true when the loss is caused by an organic condition that can be treated but not cured. If, in addition, the pattern of loss is one of deterioration followed by periods of stability or slight recovery, the person is even more susceptible to an anxiety reaction. He is caught between hope for recovery or at least the hope that he will retain his remaining sight, and the fear that in time he will lose whatever sight remains to him. Each time his sight stabilizes, he is confident that the condition has been arrested. Then he experiences a slight reduction of sight, and anxiety reasserts itself. He is convinced that eventually he will be totally blind.

The vacillation between hope and despair is perhaps the most difficult or painful pattern to cope with. The uncertainty of the outcome keeps the feelings in a state of flux, but the possibility of eventual blindness is the basis for fear. In any event, it is reasonable to assume the presence of anxiety whenever the visual condition of the client is unstable.

Anxiety that stems from the fear of total blindness cannot be relieved by false assurance regarding the outcome of the condition. The person can better be helped to understand the basis for the fear by counseling or therapy. Also, training will demonstrate that even if he should lose the remainder of his sight, he need not be helpless.

One client expressed the conflict this way: "I can't let myself believe that I won't keep the sight I have left. I believe that if I really thought I would lose the rest of my sight, I'd give up." However, later in the same session, he admitted that the basis for this assertion was his fear that he would be completely dependent on others if he lost the remainder of his sight. He also admitted that, in all likelihood, his fear of becoming dependent would motivate him to do whatever was necessary to regain his independence if he became blind.

If the visually impaired person acquires the means of dealing with the danger, he can reduce his anxiety. He can learn to do the task for which he feels he needs help, and realize that he is not helpless. He needs to understand that with no sight at all, he can perform tasks just as well as he does right now with minimal vision. In fact, he is relying to a great extent on his other senses, even if he is still using his remaining sight.

HOW THE FAMILY CONTRIBUTES TO ANXIETY

Whatever anxiety a person experiences after losing his sight can be greatly magnified by the reaction of the family. Overprotection is the most common error committed by family members when someone in the family loses his sight. Individual family members often feel that the visually impaired person is incapable of doing anything for himself. They anticipate his every wish or need. If he attempts to do even some simple thing for himself, they are quick to do it for him.

Without being consciously aware of what they are doing, they are, in fact, stimulating his anxiety. By their words and actions they imply that if he does something without help, he might injure or endanger himself. They are demonstrating to him that they believe he is helpless.

This tendency is particularly harmful during the early phase of adaptation to the loss of sight. If the person's loss has been severe enough, he is uncertain of his movements. If he attempts to walk by himself, he occasionally bumps into objects. For this reason he already feels some anxiety whenever he moves from one place to another. If at this time, some family member frequently reminds him that he is in danger, his fear increases.

If, however, family members speak quietly with a simple "stop" and then explain or indicate the proper direction he should take, no harm has been done. But if, by the effect in their voice they indicate their fear as, "Stop!" or "Watch out!" with a loud shout, the visually impaired person responds with a surge of anxiety. The increased anxiety he experiences may prevent him from making further attempts to find his way around the house. At the very least, the task will be more difficult for him emotionally.

Many families are so fearful that the blind person may injure himself that they forbid him even to attempt to cook. They worry that he might burn himself or cut himself with a knife. They may not be aware that many totally blind persons cook and do it quite safely. Often, however, they discount such information because they do not feel it applies in their situation. Thus, the warning of the family — added to the blind person's anxiety — immobilizes him. He is all too willing to listen to the family and let someone else do for him.

The same mechanism is at work when the visually impaired person takes a few tentative steps in the direction of exploring his environment. Family members warn him even about walking up and down the block and follow him to be sure he is safe. The presence of mother, father, husband, or wife constantly reminds him that some chance obstacle could present a danger. In many cases such behavior stimulates anxiety in the visually impaired person, so that he contents himself with sitting around and waiting for whatever help he can get. Of course, there are many families who do not behave in this manner. But if the behavior occurs, it usually interferes with the visually handicapped person's willingness to become involved in training toward ultimate independence.

CHAPTER 8

DREAD OF ABANDONMENT AND HOSTILITY

ABANDONMENT

Abandonment implies the previous existence of a relationship which had some meaning for the individuals concerned. It gratified some need or desire for one or both of the participants. Abandonment is then, the cessation or termination of the interaction or relationship. For some reason, one of the participants severs the relationship and the other is forced unwillingly to accept the new situation.

Abandonment is not necessarily the physical withdrawal of the significant person from his partner or sharer in the relationship. It can be just as complete and just as devastating if the significant person withdraws his emotional support. That is, he withholds love and affection that is essential to the well being of the dependent person. The significant person may be unaware that he is not meeting these needs. He may not be withholding the emotional support consciously and deliberately. The needy or dependent person in the relationship is aware that formerly his needs were met. At some point in the relationship, however, there is a noticeable change. The significant person may still be physically present, but his behavior or effect has changed. In some way, he is different. Possibly, he no longer attempts to communicate his ideas and feelings. He seems to be aloof and cold. He withholds the encouragement that may be desperately needed. He simply leaves the dependent person to his own devices.

This noticeable departure from the former and normal relationship can stimulate severe anxiety in the dependent person who interprets the change as abandonment. He attempts to reduce the anxiety by reinstating the former condition. When his initial efforts fail, he becomes frustrated because he is unable to cope with the new situation. Anger grows out of the frustration and he retaliates against the significant person. He lashes out in his attempts to regain some measure of his former security. These attempts usually fail, and when they fail, he may react with depression.

DREAD OF ABANDONMENT

Dread of abandonment is a condition that begins early in childhood and persists throughout life.[10] It stems from the helpless and dependent state of the child. He cannot feed or clothe himself and must be protected from dangerous or potentially harmful situations.

One obvious implication of this situation is that the helpless child is dependent on a particular person or persons. Because of the special nature of the helping-dependent relationship, these persons are invested with special significance by the child. They are important to him because his survival and the gratification of his needs depend on them. At some point the child becomes aware that he is dependent and that the care and protection could be withdrawn. Once he becomes aware of such a possibility, he develops the fear that he may be abandoned. As the child begins to reciprocate the love or affection he receives from the significant persons in his life, he develops an emotional as well as a physical dependence on them. Thus, whatever affection the parents show evokes a similar response from the child. Now he gradually becomes aware that if he does not respond appropriately, this affection may be withdrawn.

Normally the child discovers or learns some means of coping with the problem. He either resolves his feelings over a period of time or he develops some pattern of behavior that appeases the persons who satisfy his needs and stimulate the dread. The child may attempt to resolve the feelings of dread by the use of mechanisms such as denial, projection, or identification. On the other hand, he may mold his behavior in accordance with the parents' wishes. He may become totally compliant and be looked on as a cooperative, obedient child. Alternatively, he may demonstrate angry, aggressive behavior that is a means of testing whether or not he will be abandoned. Although the dread of abandonment may incapacitate the child or elicit behavior that is not in his best interests, it also can be the basis for developing independent behavior. The child, in conflict between his dependence and the dread of abandonment, learns that as he becomes more independent, his anxiety is reduced.

Whether the child uses some defense mechanism or develops a behavior pattern that helps him to resolve his feelings of dread, these means are at his disposal whenever he encounters a situation that stimulates the old dread. Whatever means he found to be most successful in dealing with the dread as a child are the ones he is most likely to use when, as an adult, he again experiences such dread.[10]

BLINDNESS AS A STIMULUS
FOR DREAD OF ABANDONMENT

If, as Rochlyn states, the dread of abandonment persists throughout life, it is reasonable to suppose that whatever conditions most nearly approximate the helpless and dependent phase of childhood will reawaken the dread of abandonment. One event that meets this criterion is the onset of severe visual impairment or blindness.

The sudden and severe loss of sight is usually accompanied by a state of helplessness and dependency. The degree of dependency, will, of course, be determined to some extent by the degree of visual loss. Thus, the person who retains travel vision would not, under normal circumstances, be as dependent as the person who has lost all his sight. In fact, the newly blinded person is often disoriented. Until he develops a measure of competence, he usually requires someone to guide him and protect him from potentially harmful situations. In addition, he may require help in clothing himself and preparing his food.

Although the newly blinded person may not be aware of the parallel, his situation is similar to the experience of childhood. It is as a newly blinded and helpless person that he may experience again the dread of abandonment. Although he may wish to deny the fact, he is helpless and dependent on others. The more assistance he receives, the more he is aware of how dependent he is on the one who is helping. Implicit in this arrangement, as in the case of the child, is the possibility that at some time the help might be withdrawn. The significant person could leave him: he could be abandoned. Accompanying this possibility are all the feelings that were present when, as a child, he experienced the dependency and dread. He must bring all his coping mechanisms to bear on the problem. He must resolve his feelings and learn to deal with the significant person on whom he is dependent.

The responses of some individuals may be adequate. The responses of others, however, may be inappropriate and self-defeating. In either case, they were developed in childhood. They may be ineffective, but they are familiar and the individual will continue to use them until, through some intervention he develops a more appropriate method of dealing with his dread.

Case History — Betty

Betty is a fifty-six year old woman who came to the agency while in the process of losing her sight. Her sight had been decreasing gradually over a period of a year. One year prior to her first contact with the agency, she had experienced a severe reduction in sight. She still retained minimal vision, but was severely handicapped with regard to household duties and traveling ability.

limitations due to visual loss . . .

She was married and had three married children. Her relationship with her husband, however, was extremely poor. She had experienced recurring periods of depression which became acute after her major loss of sight. The loss of sight was extremely difficult for her because of the marital situation. In addition, she had been an amateur artist and keenly felt that loss. She also found it very difficult to cope with her inability to travel freely.

marital problems prior to visual impairment . . .

In addition to the acute depressive reaction, the dread of abandonment was an outstanding feature of her reaction to the loss of sight.

Although there was no apparent emotional attachment to her husband, she was physically
very dependent on him. She needed help in
traveling and was unable to perform many of her
household duties, such as cooking. She dreaded
the possibility of total blindness, since this
would mean total helplessness and dependence.
Since she had difficulty in making and keeping
friends, she was unusually dependent on her
husband. Apart from her painting, she had few
outside interests. As the result of her visual
condition and the attendant difficulty in traveling, contact with her children and grandchildren was minimal.

dependency leading to dread of abandonment . . .

Her husband contributed to the dread she experienced by his hostile and cruel treatment of
her. He would ridicule her with comments such
as, "You think you have friends, but they laugh at
you." Such comments contributed to her feeling
of devaluation and reinforced her belief that if
her husband left her she would have nowhere
else to turn. At one time, she stated, "Having a
bad marriage and being blind is bad enough, but
living alone and being this way could be worse."

anxiety over further loss . . .

behavior contributing to dread . . .

Counseling, however, produced a marked
change in the feelings and attitudes of this
woman. She described one incident in this way:
"We were arguing and I became hysterical. I said
things I had never been able to tell him. I guess I
shocked him because I'd never acted this way
before." She also began to gain new awareness of
her qualities as a person. At one club meeting
she attended, one of the male members informed her that she was a very attractive woman.
This pleased her and added to her growing self-
esteem. She also realized that she had been
blaming herself for things for which she was not
responsible. For example, if her husband became angry when she could not read him a
phone number for which he had asked, she

growing self-esteem . . .

objectivity concerning limita-tions . . .

realized it was not her fault that she could not see the number. Betty also began making tentative efforts to begin new social contacts. Although she experienced considerable anxiety, she began traveling on city buses to visit her family. If her husband refused to take one of her talking books to the post office, she would walk to a corner mail box and deposit it herself.

Near the close of the treatment, she prepared a Thanksgiving dinner at her daughter's house. This had been her first attempt at such a task since she had experienced her major loss of sight. She had gained enough strength to tell her husband he was welcome to come if he wished, but if not, they would have dinner without him.

The greatest fear for this woman had been that when she was helpless and dependent she would be abandoned. She would have no way to initiate new contacts. This fear diminished as she became assured of her worth as an individual and as she learned that, in spite of anxiety, she could still function with her limited vision. In addition, she became confident that even if her husband abandonded her, other persons appreciated her and would not abandon her.

dread of abandonment diminishes as independence grows . . .

DREAD OF ABANDONMENT
AS CAUSE FOR MISINTERPRETATION

The newly blinded person may consider any activity that takes the significant person away from him to be a threat to the stability of the relationship. The various family members must, of course, continue with their normal activities. They cannot devote all of their time and energy to the care of the individual with a severe visual impairment. However necessary or important the activity may be, it is often apart from the routine of the visually impaired person. He is acutely aware of his inability to participate in these various activities. For him, they constitute a disruption of the relationship, since they do not include him. In fact, the blindness is in itself sufficient cause for this fear, since it disrupts the normal interaction between himself and the other family members. Thus, he observes with anxiety the involvement of the significant person in an activity of which he cannot be a part.

He interprets this as an exposure to danger. The danger is the gradual or sudden withdrawal of the significant person from the relationship. As this happens, he is convinced that it is the beginning of a process culminating in his abandonment.

DEPENDENCY

Rochlyn states, "The child pays for the security of his parents' protection by the fear of losing his parents' care and love which he tends to equate . . ."[10] The equation of love with care may be the basis for the demands of many blind persons on parents, husband, or wife. They demand special care as proof that these persons love them. The mechanism is self-defeating, however, because the greater the demands and the more they are met, the more the blind person's belief in his helplessness is reinforced. He becomes convinced that he is and will remain helpless. He sees himself as being completely dependent on the significant person. This situation stimulates to an even greater degree the fear that he will be abandoned.

FEAR OF THE DARK AND DREAD OF ABANDONMENT

Fear of the dark and fear of abandonment are present in childhood and are related. In the dark, children are separated from their parents. The environment is quieter, shapes are indistinct, and the child fantasizes more freely. It is then that he fears that when he wakes he will have been deserted by his parents. In the dark, the blurring of vision signifies lesser control of the environment. The attempt to remain awake is a mobilizing of effort to maintain control.

William stated that he had always been afraid of the dark and still keeps a light on in the hall or in the bathroom. Immediately after volunteering this information, he commented that he was afraid his wife of four years would leave him. He said that he expressed these fears to her and she assured him she would not. He is very depressed and quite helpless. His wife helps him to dress, although he says she does not baby him. To this man, losing his sight means that he will always be in the dark, of which he is afraid. His helpless and vulnerable condition stimulates the dread of abandonment.

THREAT OF ABANDONMENT BY FAMILY MEMBERS

The threat of abandonment is a potential weapon in the hands of family members who can use it to shape the behavior of a blind person. One family member may wish to keep the blind person in a dependent state because of his own need for control. Another may wish to push him prematurely into a program of rehabilitation, because the sight of a helpless person arouses his anxiety. The newly blinded person is vulnerable whether or not the member of his family is aware of this fact. In an attempt to control, he may threaten to leave if the blind person is, or seems to be, intractable. In either case, the weapon is the threat of abandonment.

In a more subtle way, a family member may simply take every opportunity to remind the blind person that he is helpless. For example, if the blind person fumbles or spills liquid from a glass, he will comment, "You should have let me help you." Or if the blind person insists on doing something for himself and fails, the family member may say, "Next time don't bother to ask me for help." A further comment may be, "You don't appreciate what I'm doing for you." First remind the blind person of his helpless and vulnerable condition; then threaten to abandon him. The withholding behavior suggests that this is just a taste of what it will be like when he is alone. Even a small dose of such treatment will have a tremendous effect on a person who already feels helpless, useless, and worthless. It adds to his feeling of devaluation and reinforces passive behavior.

Alternatively, family members may resent the dependence of the newly blinded person. They may refuse to accept the responsibility of caring for his needs. To them, these needs are a burden they are unwilling to assume. In fact, they wish to abandon the blind person and it is this wish that is evident in their communication. Through words and actions they convey their desire, even if they do not express it explicitly. The dread that this behavior stimulates is thus a realistic fear. It is not merely a function of the blind person's feeling of inadequacy or a reaction to the presence of unacceptable wishes and feelings.

THREAT OF ABANDONMENT
IN AGENCIES FOR THE BLIND

The interaction between blind persons and agencies who serve them often incorporates some element of dread and threat of abandonment. Many blind persons are regular and long-time clients of such agencies. Some of them have left normal society and have joined a group in which they feel comfortable and accepted. They are committed to this group and are painfully aware that they have no other alternative. The effort to rejoin the larger community requires too much anxiety and expenditure of emotional energy. They do not feel equipped to cope with what seem to be insurmountable obstacles. They are literally in the position of the young and helpless child who has nowhere else to go. They are, therefore, particularly vulnerable. Because they know this, they become passive and compliant. Agency personnel and administrators also know that the clients are vulnerable. They often use their position of authority to mete out rewards and punishments. The power of the agency administrator lies in the explicit or implicit threat of abandonment.

Agency administrators may not realize why their actions are so effective. A student or client who complains too much, or who knowingly or unknowingly breaks a rule of the agency is called in for a discussion. If he does not exhibit proper contrition, he is warned that if his behavior persists, he will be asked to leave. An occasional incident such as this is sufficient to perpetuate the dread of abandonment among the regular students. Students may nurture this dread among themselves, since within many of them is the knowledge that if they are dismissed, they will be alone. They may be almost totally without social contacts. Once the possibility of dismissal has been established, the dread of abandonment is implicit in the total interaction between clients and agency personnel. It does not require verbalization.

ADJUSTMENT AND RESOLVING FEELINGS OF DREAD:
Positive Aspects of Dread

In a limited way, the dread of abandonment can have positive effects, and can be a stimulus for appropriate action. If the newly blinded person feels helpless and vulnerable, he experiences anxiety at the possibility of abandonment. This anxiety, however, when combined with knowledge of the independence that can be regained through training, can motivate him. If the anxiety is too great, it will interfere with his objectivity and his ability to function. If, however, the anxiety is within manageable proportions, he can use it to turn his hope and energy to positive action. It is then a realistic means of coping with dread of abandonment.

RESOLVING DREAD
THROUGH THE ACQUISITION OF SKILLS

The possibility of abandonment is frightening and devaluing. No one likes to think of himself as being so unworthy that he can be abandoned. Therefore, the thinking of the newly blinded person gradually turns to the idea of being, in a sense, refound and taken in.   This line of thinking increases his self-esteem. He must become confident of his worth as a blind person. Even more, he must become convinced of his worth as an individual, regardless of his physical condition. The process is facilitated as he relearns old skills or develops new ones; it is confirmed as he becomes aware of his renewed independence.

HOSTILITY

Case History — Steve

Steve is a thirty-eight year old man with a wife, and two children in their teens. He had been losing his sight gradually for approximately two

*years, but in the three months prior to his appli-
cation for services, his sight began diminishing
quite rapidly. Although he had some income
from social security disability and an insurance
premium, his wife had to take a job to supple-
ment their income. In his first interview he
denied that he had experienced any strong reaction to the loss of his sight. The second
session, however, was quite illuminating:*

P: *"What has the doctor told you about your
sight?"*

C: *"He hasn't told me much of anything . . . how
fast it will progress . . . how long it will last.
But (with irony) of course he can see."*

P: *"How have you been getting along at home?"*

C: *"I'm irritable. I'm snapping at everyone. My
son says something and I bite his head off."*

P: *"Last week you told me about a friend who
tends to be overprotective. Could you tell me
a little more about that?"*

C: *"I guess I resent the fact that he complains
about his problems so much. I'd like to trade
my problems for his any day."*

P: *"Do you have any idea why you're so angry?"*

C: *(pause) "I guess it's a substitute for weeping."*

Hostility as a reaction to the loss of sight is most likely to be
displayed during the early period following the loss. It is during
this time that the person is experiencing the greatest stress.
Under the pressure of his emotions he often gives in and expresses what he feels. However, the initial period after the loss
of sight is not the only time hostility may be present. If the
individual has never resolved the feelings stemming from his
loss, the hostility may become an integral part of his personality.

The visually impaired person may express his hostility in
many ways. He may be constantly irritable or give vent to outbursts of rage for which there is no apparent provocation. Or,
he may become disproportionately angry when he accidentally

bumps himself or fails to find something for which he is searching. He also may express hostility in the form of ready sarcasm or subtle humor, which he uses to depreciate his associates or family members. The content of his remarks may have the appearance of innocence, but his comments are motivated by hostility.

It is possible, of course, that overt hostility always has been a part of his makeup. The added stress resulting from loss of sight undoubtedly will increase his anger. In addition, his hostility may change from ordinary sarcasm to a more open and direct form. If, however, the person has been easygoing, with a calm disposition, it is safe to assume that the new display of anger is directly related to the loss of sight. The emotional stress must have an outlet, and in many cases, it is expressed in anger. It may or may not be justified as it is directed toward a particular person; but it is an indication of the stress under which the person is functioning. He is, in a sense, striking out in response to the blow that he has received.

HOSTILITY AS CAUSE FOR DREAD OF ABANDONMENT

Hostile or aggressive feelings that stem from the loss of sight may give rise to thoughts such as, "I am blind and *he* can see," or "I wish *he* were blind and *I* could see." Since such thoughts are usually not in keeping with the self-image of most persons, they are threatening and produce feelings of anxiety. For this reason, they may be disguised or displaced to objects that are less worthy, such as inmates of a prison or a mental institution, or others who are considered to be useless members of society. The blind person may rationalize these feelings because certainly he can contribute more to society than any of these persons could or would. "Why should something as valuable as sight be wasted on such worthless individuals?"

Although these thoughts may be disguised or lie beneath the surface of consciousness, they actually may be directed toward significant persons such as family members or close friends. These are normally unacceptable thoughts and are felt to be deserving of punishment. For the person with impaired sight, the greatest punishment is abandonment, and this is what he fears.

GENERALIZED ANGER

Although the dread of abandonment is usually expressed in terms of loss of a significant person, it may become a generalized fear. Thus, the person may fear that he will be abandoned by society. His anger is then likely to be directed toward all sighted persons. He feels resentment toward many people who do not treat him as he thinks he should be treated. For example, they may not gratify his desire to be dependent. Therefore, because of his anger and resentment, he expects to be rejected or abandoned. As in the case of the child, he looks for a surrogate object to fill his need for belonging. Often a blind person will look to other blind persons to gratify this need. He identifies with them and finds his security within this group.

DREAD OF ABANDONMENT AS A BASIS FOR HOSTILITY

Where dread of abandonment is present, the individual will necessarily react to it, or attempt to cope with the dread in his own way. The afflicted individual may become very compliant, will go to almost any lengths to avoid antagonizing the significant person. He will then tend to become extremely cooperative, often to the exclusion of satisfying his own needs. Such a person will make almost no demands on others because he fears that asking for favors may precipitate the abandonment.

This unwilling subservience motivated by the dread of abandonment can generate tremendous anger, which may be expressed openly. Sometimes an angry outburst on the part of the blind person seems to be out of all proportion to the apparent provocation. The strength of the reaction is, in reality, motivated by the dependency and dread that the blind person is experiencing, and is not simply a function of the superficial circumstances of the moment. Of course, when such an outburst occurs, it further stimulates the existing dread.

If the blind person is unable to express his anger, this will be turned inward. He cannot satisfy all his needs because he is assuming a subservient role — he feels anger toward the person to whom he is giving precedence. In turn, he feels guilty because of these unworthy thoughts, and he believes that if the significant person becomes aware of his thoughts, he will be abandoned in retaliation. Furthermore, he feels that he deserves to be abandoned because he is ungrateful. This combination and interaction of anger, guilt, and dread often underlies the depressive reaction that so commonly follows the loss of sight. Another person may express considerable belligerence or anger and will make many demands. He will give the appearance of being perverse in his behavior.

It is less painful to withdraw from a relationship than it is to know you have been abandoned. Thus, a person who dreads abandonment may prefer to sever the relationship himself, rather than to allow the significant person to do so. It is a case of running into a feared situation versus reducing anxiety by getting the ordeal over. He also feels he has maintained control if he initiates the abandonment. In a sense he is saying, "I am the strong and worthwhile person and you do not deserve my love and loyalty." If, on the other hand, he has been abandoned, he feels that his thoughts about himself as a worthless object have been confirmed, and that the significant person is the strong one who did not need the relationship. In other words, "You are strong and do not need me. I am insignificant and worthless."

The underlying basis for the provocative behavior may again be the dread of abandonment, or the anxiety aroused by the helpless condition. The person expects to be abandoned; therefore, he behaves in a way calculated to precipitate the situation he fears. Thus, in a perverse and self-destructive way, he has maintained control of his destiny. He has used this means to reduce his anxiety. He has not been abandoned, but rather feels that he has rejected the significant person.

CHAPTER 9

FRUSTRATION

When an individual first loses all or a major portion of his sight, he discovers that he is living in a perpetual state of frustration. The frustration may occur when he can no longer function as he formerly did, and it may result when he is blocked from achieving his goals. It may come because he is bored by his enforced inactivity; or it may be due to the reduced stimulation that is an inevitable consequence of the loss of a major sense. Whatever the reason for his feeling of frustration, he must learn to cope with it. He must work toward resolving the feelings that stem from the facts of his condition.

The person with sight experiences his own share of frustration. Undoubtedly, he will do things or fail to do things that stimulate the feeling. He may mislay his glasses and spend frustrating minutes searching for them before he can read the morning paper. He may forget where he saw the garden rake or some other tool and feel frustrated because he is spending time looking for them during which he could be performing an already disagreeable task. Or a file folder with all the information needed for the next appointment may not be in its proper place in the filing cabinet. Of course, we would probably all agree that such frustrations result from simple carelessness, ". . . maybe mine, but probably yours."

Looking for the object may be frustrating, but usually the period of frustration can be limited, With sight, it takes only a few moments to scan a room for a pair of reading glasses. "Either the car keys are on the kitchen sink where I thought I left them, or they are on my wife's dresser where she must have moved them when she straightened up the kitchen."

Without sight, such a task might seem monumental. "I have to use my hands to feel all over a table or dresser top when looking for some object. Even after searching in all likely places, I can't be sure I haven't missed the item by just a few inches. So I must begin searching all over again. If a sighted person is in the house, I can ask for help. But this course presents other problems. If I must ask for help, it reminds me that I am dependent on another person. Not only am I reminded of this fact, but I am angry at the person who moved the object . . . and the person to whom I go for help may be the very one who moved it. The intention need not be malicious; the item was simply in the way and it was moved. However, I do know it was moved, and I become progressively more frustrated until I find it or ask for it."

"When I could see I would occasionally drop an object such as a coin, a bottle cap, or a pin. With no particular difficulty I could watch its progress as it bounced or rolled across the floor. I might experience some frustration in searching for it if it were quite small or if its color were the same as the surface on which it dropped. Now that I cannot see, I must depend on my hearing and touch to find what I drop. If I drop a coin, I must stop what I'm doing and listen carefully to orient myself to the position of the object by the sound it makes. Possibly I find it with one sweep of my hand. Sometimes, however, the object rolls silently for some distance before it stops. At another time, I drop an object on a rug where it makes no sound. In either case, I must get down on the floor and spend time feeling for it. In another case, I drop several coins at the same time. They roll in different directions and I feel frustrated trying to decide which to listen for, since I cannot accurately follow several sounds moving in different directions at the same time. In other situations, other sounds may mask or block out the sound of the object I am looking for. My only real choices are to forget about what I would like to find, search until I find it, or until I reach my level of tolerance and ask for help."

Many of the problems I have described can be resolved through training, practice, and the use of memory. However, the person who has recently lost his sight has not had the opportunity to adapt and to cope with frustration. Instead, he is left in the predicament of attempting to cope with a frustrating situation without adequate tools for doing so. It is no wonder then, that in his frustration, he spends so much time comparing his present limitations with his former ability to function.

REDUCTION IN STIMULATION

"When I could see, there were many experiences to attract or engross me. While driving a car or riding in a train there was the flow of passing scenery to occupy me. There was the constant shifting, blending, and separation of near and distant objects. There was contrast and similarity in the changing panorama. If I were a passenger and I became bored with the scenery, I could pick up a book, newspaper, or magazine and give my attention to the printed material as a diversion. With sight there was availability, variety, and choice in the opportunity for mental stimulation. If my interest was in physical activity, I again had the opportunity for variety and choice. I could hike in the mountains — walk or run. I could participate in or observe various sports. Now I cannot see, or at best, I see only a little. As a passenger in a car or on a train, for me, the scenery is either non-existent or a meaningless blur. Time drags, but I cannot pick up a newspaper or magazine, because I cannot read. I must anticipate and prepare for such times or expect to be bored. If I have learned to read braille, I can take along some braille material. If I have not yet learned this skill, I must be locked into my own thoughts, unless I have a companion who is willing to talk. Sitting at home and listening to the radio might seem an adequate pastime, but listening to the same program day after day can be boring and frustrating because the activity lacks variety. Furthermore, if I do find a television program I can enjoy, and the conflict is resolved within the last minute of the show in a silent scene, I am left feeling frustrated, because to me there has been no resolution. It is possible to get books on records (talking books), but if I am newly blinded, I may not know about this service. Even if I use it, I am still deprived of the visual stimulation which was a large part of my experience prior to my loss of sight. I am unaware of how my environment looks."

This frustration stemming from boredom or lack of activity is one of the most common complaints of persons who have recently lost their sight, and who have not yet acquired the means for new sources of stimulation. Without help, they find it difficult to solve this problem. They talk about things they do as though they can still see. They describe a recent trip in the language of sight: "You should have seen those mountains. They were really beautiful." "You should have seen that fish jump. He got away, but I'll swear he was the biggest one I ever hooked. He was at least *this* long." "As soon as I saw that dress, I knew it was the one I wanted."

A whole range of experiences is eliminated with the loss of sight. "I still feel and hear; I still think and know, but what I think and know has been affected by what I have lost. My visual experience remains only in memory." "If a friend describes something to me, it may evoke a remembered experience. But I am not experiencing something new or fresh. The description and the memory may be interesting and pleasant, but it is only a substitute for the real experience. The description of a visual event can never be as real and stimulating as the actual experience of seeing. I know this and because the experience is limited, I feel the frustration *because* I cannot see for myself."

LACK OF ACTIVITY

The loss of sight greatly reduces physical activity. This will be influenced to some extent by how much sight the individual has lost and how willing his friends are to help him remain active. Furthermore, the training he receives will shorten the time in which he is greatly restricted, and expand the possibilities for his becoming active again. If the individual retains some sight, he still will be able to take walks without assistance. Even if he is totally blind, he can learn to travel if he receives proper mobility instruction. If his family and friends are willing to include him in their activities, he may find many things to keep him occupied.

However, there will always be some things that a visually impaired person can never do, or can do only with help, because he cannot see. He might have sight enough to play with cards that are larger than normal, but he needs the cooperation of family or friends if he is to use these special aids. If he is totally blind, he must use braille cards; and he cannot learn to read braille overnight, contrary to some of the myths promulgated by certain television shows. If he enjoyed browsing through the stacks in a library or a book store, he can no longer do so without help. The freedom and convenience of driving a car may have been a real pleasure, but without sight, it is an unwise pastime. He may have enjoyed an occasional game of billiards, but billiard balls are not usually lettered in braille. Even if they were, he would not be sure of their position after the first shot.

All of this means that he must give up many things he used to do. He can substitute some activities, but this takes time and effort. If he cannot substitute or has not received adequate training to provide his own new activity, he can only sit at home and live with his boredom and frustration. This is the complaint of many persons who have recently lost their sight. They have not acquired necessary skills. They don't know what is available or possible as an alternate activity to their former interests. Above all, they are dependent on a family member or friend to provide some meaningful activity in which they can participate. In the words of one such person, "I'm bored out of my mind." The dilemma for such a person is that he can see no way out of his difficulty. He has lost his means of remaining active and enjoying his surroundings. His activity — and with it, his environment — has been restricted.

BLOCKING OF GOALS

An additional but frequent source of frustration for the visually handicapped person is the thwarting of his goals. "I am looking for a job and am told time and time again by employers or personnel in rehabilitation agencies that there are no jobs available." "My hopes are aroused when I am accepted into a job training program. I am disappointed and frustrated when I complete the training and find that I am still not able to get a job." "I need to go shopping, but I cannot go by myself because I have not yet learned to travel independently." "I want to go someplace today, but find that the people who usually help me are busy, so I sit at home and stew." "I am a young person and would like to date, but no one seems to want to go out with me." "I am elderly and feel a strong desire to be with people, but have no way to get to a senior citizens' club meeting." In every case the person has been blocked from reaching a goal. He tries over and over again until, in sheer frustration, he gives up. He might not feel that he is making excessive demands. He is only asking for the things he wants and needs to make his life tolerable.

Frustration is no stranger to any living being. It is a shared experience. But when anyone has a handicap such as blindness or severe loss of sight, it is difficult not to blame the handicap as the source of the frustration. Obviously, any handicap, whether blindness, paraplegia, or emotional instability, limits a person's ability to function. There are certain things that such a person simply cannot do or can do only with great difficulty. However, there are other frustrations that are unrelated to the handicap. The problem for the handicapped person is to determine which things stem from his condition and which are caused by the circumstances of his life apart from his condition.

During the early period following the loss of sight, it may be quite difficult for the person to isolate these factors. Many things that first cause frustration no longer do so after his feelings are resolved. Since he cannot be objective about these frustrating factors, he obviously requires help in making the adaptation.

CHAPTER 10

SELF-CONSCIOUSNESS

Self-consciousness is a trait that is shared by many people. It has its roots as least as far back as the developmental years of childhood, and is evident in the behavior of many young children. It can be described as a characteristic in which the person is very aware of what he does, what he says, and how he looks, and is brought into play during his interaction with others. Usually, the self-conscious person expects others to criticize his behavior, so he does what he can to avoid attention. In fact, he is very critical of himself and is often angry at himself when he makes what he considers to be a blunder. As a result, he attempts to mold his behavior in such a way that others will not notice him. Conversely, he may react to his feelings by deliberately drawing attention to himself by clowning or joking, because in this way he controls the attention he receives.

The trait, however, does not stem directly from the severe loss of sight. If it is present in the individual with a visual impairment, then it was undoubtedly an integral part of his personality long before he lost his sight. However, the person who is already self-conscious prior to the loss of sight is markedly affected by his loss. The effect is usually one of heightened self-awareness because he no longer has the means that he formerly had of coping with his feelings. The sighted person who is self-conscious can easily determine if someone is observing him. If he makes what he considers to be a blunder, he can quickly look around to see if anyone has noticed. If it does not seem that anyone has, then he need not feel embarrassed. Furthermore, he can often avoid situations that draw attention to himself. The important point is that through the use of his sight he can know if he has any reason for feeling self-conscious.

The same application can be made to any feature of his appearance. If he is self-conscious, he can insure that nothing in the way he dresses will attract critical attention. He can know if he is neat and clean. A woman can easily determine if her makeup and hairdo are presentable according to her standards. A man is able to determine if his tie is straight or his socks match.

Whether the standard for the self-conscious person is one of personal appearance or of competent behavior, he is severely limited if he is also visually handicapped. His personal appearance may be quite presentable, but he does not know this. He is never sure if some awkwardness or clumsiness on his part will draw attention to himself. There are many visually handicapped persons who avoid going to a restaurant to eat because of their feelings of self-consciousness. They dread the possibility that they will spill food on themselves or drop it on the table. They are afraid they will knock over a glass of liquid. If they pick up too large a piece of salad or bring an empty fork to their mouth, they feel as though everyone around is watching their awkward performance. They would prefer to stay home rather than undergo such an ordeal.

This self-conscious reaction is especially evident during the early period following the loss of sight. Every time a person bumps into something, he is sure others notice. If he stumbles on a curb or step, he feels that he has drawn unwanted attention to himself. The fact that no one notices is irrelevant. If he is self-conscious, he expects to be watched and has no means of knowing that his actions may have gone unobserved. If he makes some initial attempts to walk with a white cane, he is certain that people are stopping to watch him maneuvering along a sidewalk or across a street. If he could see, a quick look would tell him if this were true. Without sight he can neither confirm nor deny this possibility. The person feels that almost everything he does draws attention to himself, and this is the very thing he wishes to avoid because of his feelings of self-consciousness.

Where such feelings exist, they do not operate separately from other reactions to the loss of sight. If the individual is already self-conscious, it will interfere with his attempts to learn new skills. He may be thinking more about the attention he is attracting than about what he is trying to learn. If he feels he is clumsy and that others are observing his awkward movements, the self-consciousness will add to his feelings of devaluation. If he believes that people are staring at him as he attempts to walk with a white cane, he may be inhibited and not be able to concentrate properly on the correct mobility techniques. He may even refuse to carry a cane and thus place himself in danger when crossing busy streets, because motorists do not know of his condition. He prefers to depend on his inadequate vision rather than on the identification of the white cane that warns approaching motorists of his visual impairment.

There are two specific approaches that can be taken to counteract the negative effects of such feelings. Counseling can help the individual understand how these feelings are affecting his adjustment to the loss of sight. Training can help him overcome the awkwardness he experiences when he first loses a major portion of his sight. If he resolves his feelings and understands how they are interfering with his training, he will make greater progress. As he receives proper training, he will become proficient. When he finds that he can eat skillfully and travel competently with the use of a cane or guide dog, the level of self-consciousness should diminish. In time, he will perform these skills almost automatically. They become so habitual that they are incorporated into his new self-image.

During counseling, Bill described his feelings of self-consciousness. Because he could not eat properly, he would not eat out with friends. He mentioned this problem to his landlady, who was a friendly, helpful person, and she cooked a steak and showed him how to cut it. He was so pleased with his success in acquiring this skill he began going to restaurants with his brother. His feelings of self-consciousness diminished when he realized he was no longer awkward in handling his food.

Deanne, a young woman, talked about how self-conscious she felt when traveling with a white cane while taking mobility lessons. She felt the whole world was watching when she stumbled on a curb or walked hesitantly along sidewalks. This feeling lessened as she became skilled in her travel techniques. She realized she was no longer clumsy and gave the appearance of a competent, if visually impaired, person.

The self-conscious person probably never will become completely uninhibited, since the feeling has always been part of his personality. He always may have some residue of concern that others are watching him. However, at the very least, the feeling of self-consciousness should not interfere seriously with his ability to do the things he needs and wants to do. In spite of whatever feelings remain, he will be able to regain his self-esteem and live and work in a competent manner.

SECTION III

FAMILY AND
COMMUNITY REACTION

CHAPTER 11

FAMILY OF A BLIND ADULT

Loss to the Family

"I'm so frustrated I don't know what to do. My husband was going to retire next year and we were already planning some trips. A few months ago he lost most of his sight and now he doesn't want to do anything. He says what's the use of traveling when he can't see anything. But *I* want to go. He won't invite friends over, but wants to go everywhere with me, and I never have time to myself. I do everything I can for him and it's never enough. I practically wait on him hand and foot and if I'm not fast enough, he snaps at me. Once in a while I get out by myself, but then I worry that something might happen . . . like, what if the apartment house caught fire? How would he get out? If I'm out and start enjoying myself, I think about how miserable he is and I feel guilty. My friends say I do too much for him, but if I don't take care of him, who will? Our children live a long way from here, so they can't help. I feel as though I'm headed for a breakdown if something doesn't change. God knows he must be unhappy, but so am I. Is this the way it's going to be for the rest of our lives?"

When an individual loses his sight, the entire family has lost something. They have not actually lost the person as they would have through death, but they have lost the person — or at least their image of the person — as they knew him prior to his loss of sight.

If the visually impaired person is a husband or father, the family has lost the one who does the fix-it chores around the house. The children may have lost the person who played with them in athletic activities. Above all, if he is no longer working, the family does not have an income. Thus, to whatever degree the individual is unable to function in his former role, the family has lost a husband or father. If the visually impaired person is the mother, the family no longer has her skill and ability as homemaker. She cannot run errands, do shopping, or take the children to places that require driving. If she worked, they have lost the income on which they depended to pay part of the bills or to provide a few luxuries.

FAMILY BEHAVIOR FOLLOWING THE LOSS OF SIGHT

Case History — Ellen

"I feel as though I'm a nothing. Most of my sight went very suddenly last year and now my husband treats me like a child. I want to do some housework, and before I can start, he grabs the vacuum cleaner. I want to do the dishes and he pushes in front of me and says, 'Let me do that.' devalua-
He won't let me cook because I might burn my- tion . . .
self or spill something . . . or that's what he says. When I could see, I had responsible jobs and took care of our finances. Now he won't let me have pocket money because I might lose it. So, I can't invite a friend for lunch . . . And that's another thing: he won't let me have freedom to get away from him for a little while. He acts as though he's the only one who can take care of me. I feel useless, worthless, and angry . . . and I'm depressed."

Ellen was seventy-two and had lost most of her sight from complications of diabetes. Even though she wanted to do things for herself, her husband overprotected and controlled her. She was afraid that if she lost the remaining sight, she would become helpless and totally dependent on him. Four months before she and her husband came in for counseling she attempted suicide . . .

She took an overdose of sleeping pills but left the empty container on the bathroom floor. When her husband confronted her with it, she denied what she had done but he called an ambulance anyway. Her hospital experience was such an ordeal, it became a deterrant to any further suicide attempts. "They pumped out my stomach and it was terrible. The nurses seemed angry. They wouldn't do anything for me . . . hardly paid attention to me. It was so horrible I never want to go back . . . and that's what keeps me from trying again." However, her doctor refused to take her attempt seriously and prescribed a large number of pills, even though she told him she still felt suicidal. When she asked her husband to dole out pills as she needed them, he told her if she gave them to him, he would throw them away.

During counseling, several positive factors emerged which gave her some motivation for living. Her daughter told her how much she cared and that she would support her efforts to gain some independence from her husband. The daughter also helped the client to feel useful again by asking her to babysit the grandchildren for a weekend. In addition, Ellen began thinking about entering a rehabilitation program.

Finally her husband saw a television program on guide dogs and helped her apply for her own guide dog. With the dog she no longer felt imprisoned, since she could leave the house whenever she felt like going for a walk. Eventually she demonstrated her increased motivation by finding a doctor who took her suicidal talk seriously. He prescribed the necessary medication, but not in quantities she could use to commit suicide.

conflict about suicidal wishes . . .

hostility as basis for attempted suicide . . .

family support . . .

involvement in activity . . .

remedial factors . . .

FAMILY REACTION

When a person loses his sight, the family reacts to his changes of mood as well as to his visual impairment, because the change seems to be a drastic departure from his normal behavior. How they react depends on the specific behavior of the visually impaired person, the kinds of persons they are, and the way they feel about the loss of sight. The crisis may resolve some of the problems that exist in the family interaction. The family members may suddenly find a common goal toward which they can work. However, it is more likely that the crisis will exacerbate whatever problems already exist. A marriage that is already shaky may disintegrate under the additional burden of blindness or severe loss of sight. A son or daughter who already feels alienated from parents may withdraw even more. In any event, each family member will react to the situation in his own way.

Many of the reactions displayed by the person who has lost his sight will be present in the various family members. They may not be present to the same degree, but the feelings or emotions are often similar. They feel grief over the loss and anxiety if the loss is progressive. They also feel frustration because they do not know how to help, and anger at the way their lives have been changed. If the loss is sudden, the family almost certainly will react with shock. As they watch the newly blinded person attempt to move about the house, they are afraid he will be hurt. They feel depressed, and experience devaluation because he is no longer competent.

A family member who has a poor relationship with the blind person may feel guilt for the times he has been angry with him. He may also feel tremendous resentment toward the visually impaired person for the unavoidable dependence on him during the early adjustment period. If the relationship is sufficiently tenuous at the time of the visual loss, he feels nothing more than indifference.

If there is one common fault in the behavior of the family toward the visually impaired person, it is overprotection. In overprotection, the family members provide help that the person does not need and often does not want. They not only offer help, but insist on helping when he would prefer to do something for himself. If he says he is thirsty, someone leaps up to get him a glass of water. If he attempts to move from one room to another, someone hurries over, grasps him firmly by the arm and guides him. When he walks into the house, the person helping him almost lifts him over the threshold, and opens doors with warnings to "watch out" and "be careful."

The basis for such a strong and inappropriate reaction may be extreme anxiety or it may be reaction formation. The family member may project his own anxiety onto the blind person and "do unto him as he would like to have done unto himself." He cannot imagine how anyone can function with little or no sight, and so hurries to provide all the help he possibly can.

In the case of reaction formation, the sight of a helpless person produces so much anxiety that he wants to destroy him. Of course, such thoughts are unacceptable, so he proves to himself — and incidentally to anyone else who might be watching — that he is really a kind, considerate person who is selflessly helping the helpless. When such overprotection continues long enough, it often accomplishes the original intention. That is, the blind person becomes the totally helpless person who is never able to realize his full potential. His life, if not actually destroyed, has been limited.

I wish to emphasize, however, that the mechanism of reaction formation functions on an unconscious level. The person who reacts in this way is not aware of a wish to destroy. If he were confronted with such a suggestion, he would undoubtedly be aghast that anyone could think such a thing of him. He really believes he is doing the best for the visually impaired person.

In some cases, when the relationship between two people was poor prior to the loss of sight, the sighted person will reject the visually impaired person. The rejection may be a deliberate withdrawal through divorce or separation if the two people are married. Where the situation does not involve a married couple, the sighted person simply may leave. He walks out of the house or finds numerous excuses for avoiding the visually impaired person. He stays busy most of the time.

On the other hand, he may remain in the house, but withdraw emotionally. He refuses to give emotional support. He is there, but wants no part of whatever the blind person is feeling or experiencing.

One young woman described the situation this way: "I was so depressed I just sat and cried. I couldn't stop myself. He just sat next to me on the couch and watched TV as though I wasn't even there in the room. I was trying to clean the house and cook the way I used to before I lost my sight, but when I asked him for a little help, he refused. Said that wasn't his job."

The ideal and more mature interaction is that in which the family provides whatever help is necessary, but allows the visually impaired person to do whatever he can for himself. They encourage him to acquire the necessary skills, and curtail the help they give him as he learns to take care of himself. This type of interaction is not achieved without considerable effort and willingness to learn on the part of the family. They must also have their fair share of compassion as distinguished from pity. In addition, they usually require competent and professional help, since few families come equipped with the knowledge to help a blind or visually impaired family member in an effective manner.

One couple who came to me for counseling demonstrated such maturity and understanding. The wife had lost the sight of one eye as the result of a childhood accident. They were in their middle thirties and had two teenage children when the husband lost his sight as the result of chemical burns received at the factory in which he worked. Both wife and children provided the emotional support and encouragement he needed while he was adjusting to his loss. Eventually, he entered a new occupation following a period of retraining.

Some of the critical factors in this case of good adaptation to the loss of sight were the willingness and desire of the entire family to work toward a common goal, and concern and good communication in their relationship. In addition, what the wife experienced when she lost an eye gave her some understanding of what her husband felt when he lost his sight.

CHAPTER 12

THE FAMILY WITH A BLIND CHILD

Case History — Arthur

Mr. and Mrs. M. came in for counseling concerning their son, Arthur, who had lost his sight
as an infant due to retrolentil fibroplasia. He was
twenty-five years of age and in his second year of
college.

Most of the complaints were made by Mr. M.
"He's uncooperative and inconsiderate. Won't
come to the table when a meal is ready. He listens to his radio and TV till all hours of the night,
and won't turn down the volume even though I've
asked him often enough. I've asked him not to
take a shower in the middle of the night because
it wakes me up, but he still does it." Mr. M. also
complained that his wife was overprotective of
their son. "She won't let him walk by himself or
ride buses. She even goes to school with him."

Mrs. M. is very defensive and supports
Arthur's behavior. In addition, she rationalizes
her actions with such comments as, "I don't want
him to go for walks because he might get hurt . . .
I won't let him ride buses because the bus system
is so terrible he might get lost . . . My husband
says I favor Arthur over his brother, but it's not
true. Besides, he needs more help because he's
blind . . . I don't think that he has any real prob-

87

lems except that he needs a girlfriend. He doesn't need to change in spite of what my husband says. All I want to know is — how can I help Arthur?"

Arthur

Arthur gave the impression of speaking freely when he came in for counseling. But in fact, he spoke in a vague, rambling fashion, was very defensive, and tended to be evasive when asked a direct question. He responded to any attempt to probe his feelings by digressing to some impersonal topic. He particularly avoided making any comment that might be interpreted as criticism of his parents; but occasionally, he revealed angry feelings toward them.

His father had described a mannerism of Arthur's that especially disturbed him. He informed me that Arthur often turned away from whomever was speaking to him. I first considered the possibility that the client was only disoriented. However, this behavior usually occurred when his tone and words indicated that he did not like to answer the question he had just been asked. For example, he always turned away when I pointed out his inability to travel alone. After several counseling sessions he admitted that he rarely walked even to the corner of the block on which he lived — despite eight months of travel training — and then sometimes lost his way; and then he added, "I'm not really interested in walking." At about this time he began speaking critically of his parents in a hesitant way. He seemed to be afraid that if he expressed such criticism, they might reject him. In one session Arthur stated, "There's a girl I'd like to go out with —. She reads for me. But I know she wouldn't want to go someplace where there's a bunch of blind people." He implied by his com-

*ment that she would not be interested in him be-
cause of his blindness. As before, when I attempted
to explore his feelings, his verbal responses
became confused and rambling.*

Mr. and Mrs. M.

*When Arthur's parents came in for an addi-
tional session, I suggested that their son needed to become more independent. Mrs. M. became
extremely angry and launched into a tirade
against the bus system and sighted people.
"We've got relatives who won't help." When her
husband pointed out that she was overprotective
of both children, she attacked him with comments about relatives who won't help. It was
clear that she was threatened by the suggestion
that her son could become independent. She
refused to bring her son in for any additional
appointments, even though he could have benefited.*

When a child is born blind or loses his sight at an early age,
the family experiences the event as a severe loss. They have not
lost the child, but they have lost their original expectations of
the child and their hope for his future. Suddenly they are confronted with the fact that their child will not be like other children, and the difference will be great. Either they are sure he
will be denied all the normal activities of childhood or they are
uncertain of the possibilities for him. They assume he will not
be able to run and play and that he will require considerable
help and care. Above all, he will not be able to share in the experience of seeing, which is so much a part of their life.

If the child is already old enough to run and play when he
loses his sight, the shock will be even more severe. The family
already has an image of the child as a person. Like themselves,
he is in touch with the environment through the use of his sight.
They have known him as a normal child and suddenly he has
lost all or most of his vision. He no longer seems to be the child
he was prior to his loss. The family reacts to this change in the
child they have known. In addition, they react to whatever feel-

ings the child expresses as a result of his loss.

If the child is old enough to have been using his sight in play and in contact with his surroundings, he will experience many of the feelings that the adult experiences following such a loss. If the loss occurs suddenly, the shock will be greater. If the loss is gradual, the child will not feel anxiety about total blindness, unless he cannot yet comprehend this concept. The family, however, will almost certainly experience such anxiety as they see him becoming less able to cope with his environment. Furthermore, they will struggle with hope, and search for some cure or miracle to restore his lost sight.

Another factor that influences the reactions of the parents is their lack of knowledge and experience concerning blindness or severe visual impairment. The books they may have read prior to their personal experience provide little or no information on rearing a blind child. Their reading may have been superficial because one does not expect this to happen as a personal experience. Thus, the shock they feel when told that their child will be blind is intensified by uncertainty. They simply do not know where to turn for help or information.

SPECIFIC REACTIONS TO THE LOSS

When the parents are told of their child's condition, their first reaction is shock. They have received a blow and do not know how to cope with the information. As in the case of the person who actually experiences the loss of sight, shock is a mechanism to protect them against the pain of the loss. Following the shock period, the parents usually experience a feeling of depression. This includes an element of grief or mourning for what they have lost in the child. A further element present in the depressive reaction of parents is a feeling of guilt. They feel that in some way they have contributed to the loss of sight in their child. In other circumstances parents may feel guilt over the possibility that the visual condition could have been prevented if they had been less negligent.

The reaction of the individual parent is determined largely by his own personality. If the parent tends to react with anxiety to most situations, then the blindness of the child will stimulate anxiety. If friends or other family members demonstrate pity or exaggerated concern for the welfare of the child, the anxiety will increase. If the parent tends to be a cool, emotionally insulated person, it is quite likely he will react to the child by withholding affection.

Community attitudes and values also play their part in the reaction of the family. If a parent has incorporated the prevailing attitude — that the blind person is necessarily dependent and helpless — this will be evident in his treatment of the child. If however, his values include the belief that with adequate trainin and education the child can develop into a well-adjusted and useful adult, he will do his best to provide the help and environment that will maximize this possibility.

What the parent feels concerning the thing that has happened to his child will certainly be evident in his behavior. As in the case of the family with a visually impaired adult, the most common family behavior is that of overprotection. Without sight, the child already will be limited in his motivation to explore the environment. But the parents may discourage even limited attempts toward exploration because of their own anxiety. They are so fearful that he will be hurt that they restrict him within the playpen long after he should be exploring all the nooks and crannies of the house. They do not permit him to climb because he might fall. And as he grows and gradually should be expanding his environment, they restrict him to those areas in which they can closely supervise him.

The basis for this exaggerated degree of care, as in the case of the family with the blind adult, may be reaction formation. Again I emphasize the fact that in reaction formation the wish to destroy the helpless object is unconscious. However, the excessive protection of a blind or visually impaired child promotes the very thing that it is meant to prevent. The child is, in fact, destroyed — a helpless and dependent object. He develops into an adult who has poor or distorted concepts concerning himself, his physical environment, and his social world. Because he has been inordinately sheltered, he may find himself unable to cope with the realities of the world in which he must live. If he is able to function at all, it is only with great difficulty or with considerable help.

I do not wish to give the impression that reasonable care is not desirable. The blind or visually impaired child should be protected from objects that are potentially harmful. However, this is no more than the average parent would do for any normal child. There are risks and injuries that are a normal part of growing up, and the blind child should not be deprived of this experience which he should have in common with his sighted peers.

Other parents deny the reality of the condition. This reaction is particularly likely when the child retains enough vision to give the appearance of being sighted. These parents will expect the child to do things that are, in fact, beyond his actual capability. The child will be forced to function under tremendous pressure. He will be caught between the unreasonable expectations of one or both parents and his own anxiety. The only alternative for such a child is to adopt the mechanism of denial, which is the mechanism that his parents use to cope with the reality of his condition.

Some parents are so unable to deal with the fact of a visually impaired child that they reject him. They may do this literally by placing him for adoption, or by sending him to a residential school or nursery at the earliest possible opportunity. Other parents reject the child through the mechanism of emotional insulation. He is a part of the family and they interact with him on a superficial level, but they have no close or intimate emotional relationship with him. He is part of the household, but one or both of the parents withhold the love and affection he requires to make a good adjustment to a life without sight.

All children need the warmth and closeness of a good emotional relationship. The blind child, however, is more vulnerable because without sight he finds it difficult to initiate the contact with the significant persons in his life. The child who can see knows when his mother or father is in the room and can at any time he wishes walk over and demand the attention he desires. The blind child may not know the parent is in the room unless the parent responds to him, and so he may be left in isolation, or at least in the belief that he is alone. The result of this emotional insulation of the parent from his visually impaired child is the poorly adjusted adolescent or adult. He always seems to be out of touch with the rest of the world, because initially he was out of touch with his parents.

Fortunately, there are many parents who, without prior

knowledge of the problems of blindness, seem to do the right thing. They are mature persons who manage to deal adequately with their feelings of loss, or find help in doing so. Instead of denying or avoiding their feelings, they deal with them and actively explore community resources to aid them in rearing their handicapped child. They take advantage of the special services offered. As a result, the child can proceed through normal stages of growth and development and become a useful and contributing member of society, with a good self-image and awareness of his worth as an individual.

CHAPTER 13

COMMUNITY REACTION

The sighted members of the community have some concept of what blindness means. This is usually based on limited contact with a visually impaired person. They have seen a blind person walking down the street or have heard something from someone who may have known such a person. Thus, the information most sighted persons have is based on very little experience and hearsay.

Their reaction when they meet a blind or visually impaired individual will depend on their beliefs and attitudes about the condition, their own personality, and the behavior of the visually handicapped person. If they believe the myth of the blind beggar — or its modern counterpart, that all blind people are on welfare — they will classify in this framework any blind person they meet. All too often, their response to such a person will be one of condescension.

In general, I believe that most individuals have negative beliefs and attitudes concerning those who are visually handicapped. They believe blind persons are necessarily helpless and dependent, with the exception of the person who is especially endowed as if in compensation for his loss of sight — the blind genius.

The dread of abandonment may serve as a possible explanation for the phenomena of the blind genius. Sighted persons are usually attracted to a blind person who seems to have special endowments or unusual talents. Even if not directly attracted to such a person, they may believe uncritically that these special endowments are commonplace. The sight of such a person, or the belief that this is common, helps relieve anxiety concerning possible abandonment in the event of blindness. As in the example described by Rochlyn, the aspect of higher status is emphasized and possible abandonment is overlooked. "Of course, no one who comes in contact with a person of such special virtue and ability would consider abandoning him. Therefore, if this should happen to me . . ." Such a process of thought normally is not conscious. Instead, the progression is anxiety stimulated by the sight of the helpless person, followed by an immediate defensive reaction of identification with the more acceptable image of the gifted blind person. This identification results in a reduction of anxiety. Realistically, of course, the special endowments are not compensation for the loss of sight, but derive from personality and hereditary traits which are unrelated to and precede blindness. This knowledge is not as satisfying to a sighted observer as is the special compensation belief, and is, therefore, blocked out of his system of beliefs and attitudes.

The negative beliefs concerning severe loss of sight may explain the results of a Gallup Poll.[15] When asked to rate the condition most feared by the subjects in the polling sample, most of them placed blindness next to cancer as the condition they most feared. The factor of helplessness and dependency in cases of severe loss of sight may explain this fear. It may be anxiety about being helpless that stimulates the dread of abandonment. The more helpless the blind person appears to be, the more acute is the anxiety aroused in the observer. The crucial point, then, is not necessarily the helplessness of the blind person, but rather what this helplessness represents to the observer. He could be abandoned if this should happen to him.

Another study — at a rehabilitation agency for the blind in Little Rock, Arkansas — both supported and amplified this data.[16] Individuals who were training to work with visually impaired persons were divided into three groups. One group was composed of persons who were themselves visually handicapped. A second group consisted of those who had previously had some contact with blind or visually impaired persons, while the third group's experience with blind persons had been very slight. The first two groups demonstrated almost no negative reaction to the experience of working with blind persons. In the third group, however, many experienced shock immediately after their first contact with numbers of blind persons, followed by depression. After the depressed phase, many felt repugnance toward the persons with whom they were working.

The results of these two studies may provide a partial explanation for the experience shared by many persons when they first lose their sight — which is that friends and acquaintances abandon them. In the words of one elderly woman, "When I lost my sight, my friends left me like fleas from a dying dog." It is certainly possible that in many cases the blind person himself withdraws from normal contacts, but it is more likely that the blindness is so disturbing to many sighted persons that they avoid anyone who cannot see. Contact with the newly blinded person is a constant reminder that this could happen to them. The sight of the blind or visually impaired person thus stimulates anxiety. The only way they can reduce this anxiety is to avoid the person who is the stimulus for the disagreeable feeling.

Unfortunately, this avoidance or abandonment adds to the feelings of devaluation experienced by the person who has just lost his sight. It confirms his feelings that he is no longer worthwhile. Even if he is able to maintain a semblance of the former relationship, he is quick to notice if friends do not call as often as they used to. He is only too ready to believe that this is because he is blind.

Unfortunately, when avoidance occurs, it has tragic consequences for the visually impaired person. If he is aware that he is being rejected, his adjustment becomes more difficult. Not only does he have to deal with feelings stemming from the loss of his sight, but he also must deal with the feelings resulting from his rejection. If he works diligently toward adjustment by acquiring new skills, or trains for a new career or job, he experiences new disappointment and frustration. It is as though he has received a double blow. He has lost his sight and often his hope. Then he is retrained only to find he cannot make use of his training. It is not too surprising that under these conditions he reacts with bitterness and withdraws from the community.

This is also true for the elderly blind person who may not expect to work, but who hopes for eventual re-integration. His goals are more limited, but they are the basis for his efforts to acquire new skills. If, after his period of adjustment he finds that his sighted friends are unavailable, he has no recourse but to withdraw into the segregated and narrow association of other blind or visually impaired individuals.

One related phenomenon is the tendency of some churches, clubs, or other social organizations to separate such persons into a group within the larger group. The larger group may provide them with some help and include them in the general activities, but they are primarily a distinct entity within the larger group. The effect is thus to make everyone aware of the fact that they are different because of their physical handicap. This practice is at one and the same time an offer of involvement and a restriction on that involvement.

SECTION IV

ADJUSTMENT TO
THE LOSS OF SIGHT

CHAPTER 14

FORMS OF ADJUSTMENT

When a person loses a major portion of his sight, it is by almost any definition a detrimental event. The one who experiences this loss attempts to make some adjustment or adaptation to the new conditions of life.

Some writers seem to speak of adjustment as being only a good or positive reaction. They speak of an adjusted blind person as one having certain commendable qualities such as independence, a sense of humor, and acceptance of his condition. The term *adjustment* in itself, however, does not adequately describe all possible adaptations. The adjustment may be appropriate or inappropriate. It may be economical and to the best interests of the individual and society, or it may be detrimental and potentially destructive. Adjustment is, therefore, a term that must be qualified if it is to be meaningfully descriptive.

APPROPRIATE ADJUSTMENT

The person who has made an appropriate adjustment to his blindness makes the most effective use of his remaining abilities and senses. By taking advantage of rehabilitation training he acquires the skills he needs to become competent and relatively independent. He learns to travel independently and care for his own needs in the home. After facing his loss honestly, he resolves the feelings of grief and deals with life as it is. In order to adapt he finds ways of compensating for what he has lost. Not only does he learn to live with his condition, but he helps others to feel comfortable with it. Such a person uses his abilities and natural endowments not only for his own advantage, but also for the advantage of society. If he is of working age, he tries to find work to support himself and his family. If he is an older person, he finds other ways of being productive. By taking part in social activities, he shares himself with others. He participates in community activities according to his interest. When he needs it, he accepts help, but he gives where he can. He does this because, in spite of his blindness, he is a contributing member of the community.

Case History — Wayne

(The statements of Wayne have been taken from a number of counseling sessions and indicate the progression toward appropriate adjustment.)

"Tell you about myself? Well, I'm fifty-two years old. I have a wife and three children. I've worked most of my life in administration —. I started in a management training program, changed jobs just once, and worked my way up to supervising a department for my firm. I had that job for about fourteen years . . .

"I started losing my sight about fifteen years ago. That was when I first noticed a problem, but it wasn't very bad then. It didn't really start bothering me until about five or six years ago. My sight had been going slowly, but it's been pretty stable since about that time. I can still see quite a bit, but what I see is kind of spotty . . .

adaptation to gradual loss . . .

"Thought I was still doing a good job at work. I don't need to tell you I was pretty shocked when they terminated me six months ago. I wasn't exactly ready to retire . . . Would you believe I had to go back several times to break in the new man that replaced me? At least I didn't have to go on welfare. I was covered by insurance and I get about three-fourths pay. It's hard not to feel bitter because I really enjoyed my work . . .

shock over loss of job . . .

"My family? They've been really swell, a real help . . . I do get depressed once in a while, but

family support . . .

not as bad as when I first lost my job.

"Remember the way I used to talk against carrying a cane when I first came in to see you? I started carrying one last week. I gave it a lot of thought and decided I needed it to get around safely.

resistance followed by objec- tivity . . .

"Besides, it wouldn't be fair to any driver that might hit me if I stepped out in front of a car — because I didn't see it . . . and he wouldn't have known I couldn't see him . . .

"Someone — another blind man — told me I should hide my problem as long as I could, but I think it's better to let people know what I can see and what I can't. Otherwise, things get too con- fusing. I was tempted to take the advice because at first I didn't want people to know how bad my sight was. But it's easier for me if I can live without covering up something. I prefer to be honest about what happened to me.

advice about hiding condi- tion . . .

rejecting inappro- priate advice . . .

"I found out there are still a lot of things I can do. I always enjoyed fixing things around the house. It's really a pleasure when I find I can still do something even though I can't see what I'm doing as well. Just being able to do things is pretty important. I don't have to feel useless.

compensa- tion and growing self- esteem . . .

"I'd still like to work, but the problem with my insurance is that if I take a job, my insurance will be canceled and then if the job doesn't work out, I'm in trouble financially. I think I'll find some kind of volunteer work I can do. It'll make me feel good just to be able to help someone else. I've even learned to shoot a bow and arrow, but it's not so much fun when someone else has to tell you where to aim. I've got an idea for setting up a buzzer at the target so I can aim by myself.

"I think the hardest thing about losing my sight is learning what I can do for myself so I won't need to accept so much help from my family and other people. I never want to be a burden on them and I know now that I don't have

increasing indepen- dence . . .

*to be that dependent. Even if I lost all of my sight,
I know there are plenty of things I could do. It's
good to know that."*

INAPPROPRIATE BEHAVIOR

Inappropriate behavior is also a form of adjustment to the loss of sight. The outcome, however, is not to the best advantage of the individual or society. For example, the blind or visually impaired person may feel that he now has a legitimate way to fill a dependency need. However, he fills this need at a cost to himself and the community. He experiences a loss of dignity while the community accepts the burden of meeting his economic and social needs.

The person who has made an inappropriate adjustment might withdraw or avoid normal contacts and display relative or complete helplessness. He may be unwilling to admit the full extent of his loss. Often in such cases, he is confronted with embarrassing or dangerous situations because he is attempting to perform in ways that are beyond his physical ability.

Case History — Dennis

Dennis was totally blind when I first saw him for counseling. He had been diabetic for many years and had lost his sight as the result of complications stemming from his condition. He began losing his sight approximately five years before I first saw him, and for the past two years had been totally blind.

He was fifty-two, lived alone, and according to his statement, had no friends or living relatives. His wife had died one year after he began losing his sight. She also had been diabetic. He had never received mobility instruction and traveled nowhere without sighted help.

The dominant features of his reaction to the loss of sight were anxiety, depression, and an intense feeling of hopelessness concerning his condition and his ability to function without his sight. Whenever counseling touched on these

*feelings, he would digress to topics of less per-
sonal significance. He was, at first, very resistant in counseling and displayed a marked
tendency to mistrust almost everyone.*

The client had been a deputy sheriff prior to
the loss of sight, and expressed much bitterness
because he had been forced to give up an occupation he very much enjoyed. For a time he had
been in training as a vending stand operator, but
felt this kind of work was beneath him. He frequently expressed negative feelings about the
program and his part in it.

His contact with the agency seemed to be a
hesitant attempt to reach out for help, but he
never participated in any rehabilitation classes.
Eventually he stopped coming — even for counseling. His case is a good example of clearly
inappropriate adjustment to the loss of sight.

The following comments taken from counseling
sessions demonstrate his feelings concerning
the loss of sight, as well as his resistance to a
more appropriate adjustment.

*"I know I signed up for classes, but I'm not sure
I want to come back again . . ." "I want you to tell
me what the purpose is for my coming here to
the agency . . ." "You know, it's hard for me to
trust people. I test them by phoning and pretend-
ing to be someone else. I want to get their
reaction." "Why should I be coming to see you . . .?"
"If you would recommend it, I would have myself
committed to a mental hospital."*

resistance to rehabilitation . . .

wish to be dependent . . .

*(After talking about his former job): ". . . What
you don't realize is that my basic problem is un-
solvable. I've lost my family and I'm all alone.
Now I've lost my sight. Nothing is going to
change that." ". . . Getting into the vending stand
program was really a comedown after the work
I've been doing. Besides, they favor anyone who
still has some sight. As soon as you lose all your
sight, they don't want you anymore. I had to
swallow my pride even to go into the program."*

devaluation . . .

"*. . . You know, I don't believe that a person who has any sight at all can understand what it feels like to be blind.*" "*If you told me what to do or diagnosed my condition, I would accept it without criticism.*" "*When I say a partially sighted person doesn't understand what I'm going through, I mean it!*" "*. . . I don't believe a blind person can ever be a good traveler. I have trouble finding my way around my own apartment. Any person who claims to be blind and can get around has got to be able to see at least a little.*" "*I guess maybe I don't have any motivation to learn to travel with a cane.*"

lack of motivation due to anxiety . . .

CHAPTER 15

WITHDRAWAL AND FANTASY

One form of adjustment to the loss of sight is withdrawal. In most cases some degree of withdrawal is an unavoidable consequence of a major loss of sight. The person loses his ability to travel freely and thus, loses his initiative in making normal social contacts. If, in addition, the individual is severely depressed, he has lost his interest in normal social interaction. However, the withdrawal should be only a temporary condition. With the acquisition of travel and other skills, the individual should be able to resume many of his former activities. As he resolves the feelings that attended his loss of sight, he should regain his former interest in associating with friends or acquaintances.

Many visually impaired persons, however, who have never resolved their feelings, continue in a state of withdrawal until it becomes a habitual pattern. To such a person withdrawal has become a means of coping with an unbearable reality. He may feel lonely or alienated because of his isolation; he may be completely dissatisfied with the emptiness of his experience. The lack of mental stimulation may be extremely boring and he may feel frustrated by his enforced idleness. Nevertheless, withdrawal has become his way of dealing with the visual loss and he adheres to it because it is familiar and safe.

Withdrawal following the loss of sight may take two forms. The visually impaired person may withdraw physically. That is, he avoids all but the most essential contacts. On the other hand, he keeps up his social contacts, but withdraws emotionally from the people he knows or meets.

PHYSICAL WITHDRAWAL

In this form of adjustment the individual literally removes his presence from others. He may do this passively or actively, but he severs most, if not all, of his social contacts. Whenever possible, he hides in the familiar and secure surroundings of his home and makes no effort to contact former friends. He deprives himself of the pleasure he once felt from attending concerts or parties, or from visiting with friends. When he receives invitations to social functions, he makes excuses. If he does go out, it is only with a family member or one or two close friends. He particularly avoids new experiences in unfamiliar surroundings.

Such a person certainly has made an adjustment. He has made a compromise between his desires and his physical condition. Because he has given up so many activities and relationships, he exists in a condition that is barren when compared with his former life. In exchange, he has the relative security of his home. His family makes few demands on him. Their expectations are lowered in keeping with what they consider to be his limitations. He receives little, but gives even less.

EMOTIONAL WITHDRAWAL

In this form of adjustment the person maintains all or most of his social contacts. He still attends church, goes to parties, or attends meetings of his fraternal organization. A woman may still visit with the neighbors, go to lunch or to the beauty parlor with a friend, or attend P.T.A. meetings. Such persons go through the motions of interaction, but they scrupulously avoid any exposure of their true feelings. They interact but do not permit any closeness in a relationship. It is as if they have been sensitized to the pain of possible rejection. They are so sensitive to the difference between themselves, as visually impaired, and others, that they expect a rebuff if they reach out for emotional closeness.

These persons choose — or drift into — the security of superficiality in their relationships. They shake hands and talk about the weather; they discuss baseball scores or the latest fashions; or they talk about what so and so is doing. Often these persons hide what they really think and feel. The content of their communication is an indication that it is a defense. Their conversation is primarily a means to control the direction and extent of their communication. Someone might intrude on their privacy by offering or demanding closeness that they are afraid to give. To expose their feelings would leave them vulnerable.

As in the case of physical withdrawal, these persons are making an adjustment to a painful experience. It is their way of coping with the loss of sight and its meaning to them. Furthermore, if this form of withdrawal is a drastic departure from their former way of interacting with others, it is an unsatisfactory solution. They do not feel comfortable or natural with this behavior, and the stress they experience takes away much of the pleasure they would normally feel. They expend considerable emotional energy to maintain distance. (In a sense, they are in continual conflict between the desire for the social contact and the wish to avoid the contact.) Eventually they become so closed in to themselves that they find it difficult ever to break through the habit of isolation or emotional insulation.

FANTASY

Fantasy or daydreaming is a mental activity that everyone employs, to some extent. Even a person who is quite busy has time for an occasional daydream, while the person who has considerable leisure may spend much of it in fantasy. In addition, the person who is endowed with a rich imagination may derive much pleasure from the long periods of time he can devote to his daydreams, while the less imaginative person concerns himself with activity outside of himself. The difference between individuals is in the amount of time spent in daydreaming, as well as the quality, content, and the motivation for it.

The content of the fantasy may be constructive. That is, the person is imagining or making plans that eventually he will put into effect. In this sense, fantasy is the birthplace of great inventions, scientific advancements, or ideas for social change. Fantasy is, thus, the beginning or stimulus for action.

Fantasy can be destructive when it always stops short of action. Daydreams become a substitute for what the person really wants to do. In his imagination he does great things and enjoys pleasurable experiences, but nothing changes in his circumstances or relationships. He dissipates his emotional energy and wastes years of his life without achieveing his goals. Since he has done nothing in which he can take satisfaction, his self-esteem suffers. Much of fantasy has its beginning in thwarted goals or personality conflicts, as well as in physical limitations of the individual. The person may not be able to gratify his sexual desires because of his sexual conflicts. Anxiety may prevent him from achieving his goals, or he may be thwarted by other persons or circumstances. He may be physically or mentally incapable of doing the things he believes he would enjoy doing. Whatever the case, he is blocked from within or without from doing what he wants to do. In fact, the goals may be socially unacceptable.

FANTASY AS A SUBSTITUTE FOR ACTION

When a drive toward a particular goal is strong enough and the individual is prevented from taking direct action, he may gratify his wishes in fantasy. In this way he can achieve the goals that have been denied him in reality. The fantasy may not be as satisfying as the real goal would seem to be, but it has the advantage of being unrestricted. It is, thus, an easy replacement for an unattainable reality. The content of the fantasy may be aggressive in character or it may be entirely harmless. But it is an easy substitute for reality. The convenience of fantasy is that it is so easily molded to meet the needs of the individual. In fantasy, everything comes out right. Everything is possible, subject only to the push and pull of inner forces.

The person who is prevented from transforming his wishes into action must have some other outlet for his feelings. For example, if he has been immobilized by blindness, he may spend much time daydreaming about what he would like to do, or reliving former experiences. He fantasizes himself actually seeing and participating in normal activity. The specific content of the daydream or fantasy is an expression of what is important or necessary to him. It is influenced by his age and special interests, or by his needs and conflicts. The daydream may be a memory or a wish, but it is shaped by his special need.

When a person has lost all or most of his sight, it is almost axiomatic that activity denied him by the loss of his sight will be uppermost in his mind. He wants to see — because without sight he is denied the gratification of many of his desires. It is an easy transference from wishing he can see to imagining that he is seeing again. In his imagination, everything is right and he is once more an independent and worthwhile person.

FANTASY AS A REACTION TO LOSS OF SIGHT

Many of the feelings that stem from the loss of sight stimulate fantasy. Fantasy is an antidote to the anxiety the person experiences when he attempts to function without being able to see. It compensates for feelings of devaluation and is a safe means of expressing the hostility he feels toward those on whom he is unwillingly dependent. Furthermore, it is in his fantasy life that he can give free rein to his grief.

Without sight, the newly blinded person does not have the means he once had to take direct action. He has not yet acquired the skills for good functioning, and he has much time on his hands. If he was a busy, productive person prior to the loss, he has a strong need to fill the mental void. Whatever hope he has may be in direct contradiction to the physical world or medical reality. It is no wonder then, that in fantasy he returns to the real experience he has lost. His physical activity — and therefore the means to gratify his wishes — has been restricted, and his fantasy is readily available to replace what he has lost.

It is often the case that a person who feels his loss greatly will exaggerate his ability in his fantasy. The image of himself as the hero in many situations is an example of such compensation. He feels strong and adequate in his fantasy because he is aware of his inadequacy. No matter what problems he encounters, he will be able to solve them in his imagination and be of help to others. Often a newly blinded peron will make the comment, "If I ever should get my sight back, I would devote my life to helping the blind." This comment could be a clue to the blind person's self-image as a hero in his fantasy life. However, it could also indicate a wish to atone for real or imagined misdeeds for which blindness is a punishment. In either case, it is worthwhile to explore the fantasy life of the person to determine the origin or motivation for the statement.

Whether or not the person with severe visual impairment voluntarily discloses his fantasies, they are a very important part of his attempt to adjust to his condition. They indicate not only how he feels about himself because of his loss, but also how he feels about the people he meets and on whom he is dependent. The more painful the loss, the more restricted he feels; and the more anxiety he experiences, the more he will depend on fantasy to give meaning to his existence.

When fantasy is used as an alternative to action, it is self-defeating because it leads nowhere. The person gains only temporary relief from the bleakness of his existence. Eventually, he must face the fact that in reality, nothing has changed. He is still the helpless, dependent person he was when he first lost his sight. Unfortunately, the individual may spend months or years in the cul-de-sac of fantasy. He has spent precious time dreaming of what might have been or could be, rather than directing his emotional energy toward a real and meaningful solution to his problems. He has spent time in dreaming that could have been used learning to function without his sight. His fantasy life has been an escape from pain or frightening reality; but it has also been a withdrawal from a meaningful and satisfying life.

CHAPTER 16

DEPENDENCY

The dependent, helpless condition of the person who has recently lost his sight is in all probability the greatest contributing factor to the reaction that he experiences. It is this factor that causes the most drastic changes in his life situation. It affects his relationship with the family and friends; it changes his status in the community; and if the loss is severe enough, it makes him completely vulnerable to the demands or whims of others.

Even when there is no malicious or uncharitable intent on the part of the people with whom he must interact, he feels his helplessness. This in turn affects how he will interact with others. Every time he must ask for help he knows that he is dependent and helpless. The knowledge is a constant reminder that he is not the independently functioning person he was formerly. If his loss is severe, he is quite literally in the position of the child he once was. It is quite common to hear statements from clients such as, "Well, it's like starting all over again," or "I feel as though I'm back in school," or "You have to crawl before you can walk." This dependent and helpless condition is the basis for much of the anxiety the person experiences. It is the basis for the feeling of devaluation, and above all, it is the factor that contributes to feelings such as dread of abandonment.

Dependency in one form or another is a fact of life for everyone. No one lives or survives completely on his own initiative or resources. This is particularly true in our modern, complex civilization. However, for the person who can see it is relatively easy to maintain the illusion of independence. Because he can

113

see, he can travel with relative freedom and can believe that he is reasonably independent. In addition, because he can read signs or labels, he can more easily use the products of a modern civilization.

The person with little or no sight, however, is acutely aware of his dependence on others. Specifically, he is dependent for help and services on those who can see. His very survival depends on these people. Any attempt to convince himself to the contrary requires a well-functioning mechanism of denial. For example, he may be able to get to and from the grocery store by himself, but to find the items he wants, he needs help from someone who can read the printed material on labels. He may be able to dial a telephone number and call a doctor without help, but he must memorize a phone number given by someone else or must call the information operator for the number.

It is evident, then, that some tasks are difficult, if not impossible, for the person with severe visual impairment. But there are some he can perform without help and others which he can perform when he acquires the skill. In other words, there are some ways in which he is realistically dependent and other ways in which he is relatively independent.

FACTORS AFFECTING DEPENDENCY

One factor that affects the dependency of a visually impaired person is the degree of remaining vision. A totally blind person, of course, could read nothing. But a person with minimal sight might be able to read some types of printed material, depending on contrast, lighting, and size of the print. He could do this even though the effort might be frustrating and emotionally wearing. Furthermore, a person with reasonably good visual acuity, but greatly restricted field vision, could actually drive a car, although he would do so at his own risk or the risk of others. In fact, there are some persons classified as legally blind who still drive because the state in which they live does not require them to pass field tests of vision in order to obtain a driver's license.

A second factor in determining realistic dependency is the amount and quality of training a visually impaired person has received. If he has already undergone some training, he may have acquired sufficient skill in certain tasks to minimize his dependence on sighted persons. He can compensate through training for some tasks that are at first impossible. He can also substitute braille reading and writing for print.

A third and more critical factor is the time that has elapsed since his visual impairment. The process of acquiring new skills or relearning old ones takes time. In addition, the emotional adaptation to the loss of sight often takes months or years. However, time in itself does not bring independence. Some visually impaired persons have lived for years without developing compensatory skills, and as a result remain quite dependent on friends and family. They find it difficult to function or orient themselves — even in the familiar surroundings of their own home. Others, in a relatively short period of time following a major loss of sight, have made a good beginning toward relative independence. They may not be able to travel outside the home because they have had no mobility training, but they can move about quite well within their own home. They have learned, or at least attempted to learn, ways of caring for some of their own needs. It is, however, important to be aware that in the early stages of sudden and major loss of sight the blinded person is usually quite helpless and dependent.

UNREALISTIC DEPENDENCE

Unrealistic dependence, on the other hand, is primarily related to emotional factors. In such a case, the person may act more helpless than he is or needs to be. In fact, he may not be able to read, but he should be able to orient himself sufficiently to find the bathroom in his own home. He may not have developed the skill of dialing the telephone, but he should be able to talk to the doctor himself without depending on a family member to make the call for him. Cooking a meal may be more than he can manage, but he should be able to find what he needs in the refrigerator and fix a sandwich when he is at home alone.

If the blind person attempts to do things for himself, it indicates that his dependence is realistic. The sandwich he puts together may be sloppy, but it is something he has done himself. He may bump into a wall because he lacks adequate training in orientation and defensive techniques, but he does not wait for someone to lead him from a chair in the living room to a chair in the kitchen. Such active behavior is at least an indication that he is dissatisfied with his dependent position and wishes to develop independence.

Often the family contributes to the state of unrealistic dependence. They insist on doing almost everything for the blind person — to the point of anticipating his every need. They discourage him from attempting to move about the house without help. Through their solicitous efforts they manage to blunt the edge of whatever desire he has for independent action.

When the evidence indicates that the individual is being unrealistically dependent, it is essential to determine the basis for this behavior. It may be that his level of anxiety is so great that it inhibits his wish for independence. However, it may be that the loss of sight has provided the excuse to satisfy a wish for emotional and physical dependence. While he still can see, he defends himself against this need through reaction formation. He deliberately chooses an occupation or specific behavior that holds the dependent wishes in abeyance. He cannot allow himself to give in to his dependent wishes because as a physically normal individual such a capitulation would stimulate strong guilt feelings. The values he has incorporated would not allow him to give in to the desire to be nurtured. But without normal sight, he can allow someone to take care of him without the accompanying feelings of guilt.

One such person was a man who had been involved as a leader in a labor movement. He agitated for better conditions and led strikes and demonstrations. When he suddenly lost his sight, he became completely helpless. He was unable to find his way around his own home and depended on his wife and son to lead him from one room to another. He could not even consider the possibility that after training, he might work again. He felt that as a blind person he could never participate in his former profession.

While his behavior as a blind person seems inconsistent with his former personality traits, it is understandable. All persons have some desire — in some way or at some time — to be dependent. However, such a person as the man described had such a strong dependency need that he reacted against it by taking a strong leadership role. Acting as a dependent person would have been inconsistent with his concept of himself as a strong person.

When, however, he lost his sight, he had the excuse he needed to become the dependent person he unconsciously wanted to be. He could now be dependent and helpless without the accompanying feelings of devaluation. After he lost his sight, family expectations of him were not as high as they had been. His friends and family actually encouraged these attitudes. Therefore, because of his blindness he was able to satisfy his dependency needs.

UNREALISTIC INDEPENDENCE

Some persons react to their loss of sight by refusing help even though they need it. They attempt tasks for which they are not prepared by training. At other times they endanger themselves or others by their behavior. A typical case is a person who has not received adequate mobility training and yet refuses help when crossing a street.

Another person who is severely visually impaired refuses to carry a cane, putting himself in danger, and frightening motorists as he steps down from a curb almost in the path of an approaching auto. One elderly man who was totally blind attempted several times to back his car out of the driveway by using his cane to follow the edge of the lawn. He could not possibly have known whether or not a child was playing behind the car. While normal attempts to acquire skill and independence are admirable, such behavior is foolhardy. It is, in all probability, a reaction against the realistic dependency needs stemming from the loss of sight.

NEGATIVE ASPECTS OF DEPENDENCY

As the blind person develops capability in many areas, he finds less need to overreact to those situations in which he is clearly dependent. He can allow someone to take care of him without the accompanying feelings of guilt. Society does not condemn him in his new and dependent role as a blind person, so he need not condemn himself. Dependency, however, has certain drawbacks, especially when we have no choice in the matter. To some degree or at some time, all of us would like to be dependent. It is a holdover from the secure, comfortable period of childhood when all our needs were met. For most adults, dependency loses its appeal when it becomes total and apparently permanent. This is often the case during the early period following the loss of sight.

One of the most frustrating aspects of dependency is the necessity of waiting for someone to meet our needs — at their convenience. The other person may be quite willing to help but he is not always available at the right time. He has obligations and needs of his own. Our requests may not seem as urgent as his own needs. Thus, the dependent blind person cannot always do things when he want to — as he would if he were able to function independently. Usually, he cannot act on impulse, but must wait and coordinate his schedule with the other person's. And if he cannot obtain help, he must face inevitable disappointment. He may feel angry and frustrated because his plans have been thwarted, but he cannot express his feelings unless he is willing to risk the possibility of being rejected.

Loss of privacy and self-determination result from dependency. Since someone else must read his mail, the visually impaired person must share the information — no matter how personal it is — with the reader. He must, in addition, do this without prior knowledge of what the letter contains. When a dependent blind person wishes to do something or go somewhere, he must first share his plans with the person he is asking for help. As he shares his plans, he risks the helping person's intervention with unwanted advice or suggestions. At the very best, he expects such a reaction, even if the helping person has no intention of interfering. At the worst, he must defend his plans or intentions or give an explanation for what he intends to do. This situation usually is further complicated by the normal interaction between two persons in a dependent-helping relationship. The dependent blind person feels obligated to accept advice from a person he has asked for help. Conversely, most people feel they have a right to give advice to a person they are helping. Thus, the dependent-helping interaction places added strain on the relationship between the visually impaired person, his family, friends, or acquaintances.

The dilemma for the visually impaired dependent person is that he is rarely aware that his demands are unreasonable. The basis for his behavior may be anxiety or a need to be nurtured, but he does not know this. He justifies his requests and demands because he feels he simply cannot function without his sight.

CHAPTER 17

DENIAL AND PROJECTION

Denial and projection are the two earliest mechanisms to appear in the development of the child. They serve the child in his attempts to deal with difficulties in his relationship with his parents. In this relationship he soon becomes aware of a connection between the expression of his own angry feelings and the responses of his parents. If he directs his anger toward them, they respond with a reprimand or some more severe form of punishment. He fears this retaliation because he is dependent on them. Since the child cannot control the angry feelings, he dissociates himself from them. He denies they exist and he attributes them to the persons against whom he feels the anger. He feels his anger but says, "You're mad at me. You don't love me." Often the child uses this response in any threatening or unpleasant situation. He hurts himself on a toy but says, "It hurt me."

The person who uses denial as a mechanism conceals or distorts the true meaning of a threatening situation. Because he cannot admit the presence of anxiety, he cannot deal with the feelings. If he denies that a situation is threatening, he can neither attack it nor escape. Nor can he ever learn that, in fact, he has nothing to fear in it. Thus, he never discovers that he can improve his situation.

In the normal course of development most children learn to use more mature methods of dealing with threatening situations. If there is discord between themselves and their parents, they do not deny that they are angry or afraid, but instead, through identification, incorporate the values and code of their

119

parents. Gradually, they give up their dependence, but find ways to compensate for what they give up.

The visually impaired person may deny that his loss is as severe as the doctor says it is. He may retain only minimal sight, but insists that he has enough sight to get around quite well. On the other hand, he may accept the fact that he has lost a major portion of his sight, but insist that what he has lost is not important or worthwhile. A typical denial statement is, "Blindness is only a minor inconvenience." By this statement the person implies that what he has lost is not valuable, since he can get along so easily without it. Another way such a person can deny reality is to emphasize the minimal sight he retains rather than speak of what he has lost. He does this, not because he wishes to evaluate his remaining assets objectively, but because he cannot cope with the extent of his loss. If he faced his loss head-on, he might be overwhelmed.

Another person who uses the mechanism of denial readily admits the extent of his physical loss, but denies that the loss has any meaning for him. He might say, "So I lost my sight. It doesn't bother me. In fact, it's all very humorous the way it happened to me." By not permitting the feelings access to consciousness he is able to cope.

PROJECTION AND VISUAL LOSS

In conjunction with denial the visually impaired person often projects his feelings onto others. He can see them in another person more readily than he can in himself. One middle-aged woman, when describing her loss of sight said, "You know, the whole family really feels bad about what's happening to me. They're so upset. As a matter of fact, they feel worse about it than I do. I don't know why they should feel that way; it's not *that* bad — nothing to cry about." In this way she dissociated herself from the feelings. This is not to say that the feelings she described in the various family members were not genuine. Persons who project sometimes see in others feelings that actually exist. The crucial point is that the feelings also exist in themselves, but they deny it. Thus, her description of the way in which the family members reacted to her loss contrasted sharply with her account of her own reaction or lack of it. It is significant that she made light of what the various family members felt concerning her loss. In this way she was able to cope with what she could not allow herself to feel.

CONSEQUENCES OF DENIAL AND PROJECTION

Unfortunately, the person who uses denial as a defense often refuses services that could benefit him. If he does not believe he has lost a significant portion of his sight, he will have no reason to go to an agency for retraining. In all likelihood, he will attempt to travel without a cane when he cannot do so safely, and he might try to drive a car when he cannot see well enough to prevent an accident. This form of denial is most likely to occur when the loss of sight is gradual. As the person's sight deteriorates he will try to accommodate to the loss and convince himself he still has enough sight to perform adequately. He may not admit — even to himself — that he is making errors until he has a serious accident or until someone intervenes.

Case History — Charles

Charles, age seventy-six, came in for one counseling session because he couldn't reconcile his loss of sight with his religious beliefs. For some time he had been aware that his field vision was decreasing, but tried to ignore the change. One day, while driving he lost a major portion of his sight. Despite the sudden loss, he drove the remaining distance to his home with his wife's verbal assistance. He denied having any emotional reaction to the loss of sight, but at one point during the counseling session began crying. Charles also told me he continued to drive in his neighborhood until he was involved in two minor traffic accidents. However, he claimed that neither of these was his fault. When he finally quit driving, it was because he "didn't want to do anything foolish."

CHAPTER 18

IDENTIFICATION

When the mechanism of identification begins to develop, the child uncritically takes on the values and restrictions of his parents in order to please them. Through insight, he gradually realizes the purpose behind the restrictions and ideals of his parents. Later, he sees the affect of his actions on others and changes his behavior according to the new understanding. As he continues to mature, he identifies with children of his own age, and shares secret information with them. Through this sharing, he learns that another person who is just as afraid as he has succeeded in a difficult situation.

When he eventually identifies with a group, he can benefit. He can become stronger through sharing experience, and can accomplish things he could not do alone. Because he receives support, he does not need to feel helpless; and as a member of the group, he receives recognition.

Close identity with a group, however, may have negative aspects. The goals and decisions of the group are not always compatible with his own. The group may dominate or exploit him. It may not permit him to associate with individuals or groups of which they do not approve. Or it may even determine which thoughts and values are permissible.

It is the mechanism of identification that influences persons in their choice of a group. Those with common characteristics or shared experiences tend to come together. The similarities may be real or imagined, but if an individual believes a kinship exists, he will feel allegiance to the group. As he becomes part of the group, he will achieve a measure of self-approval. This sense of self-approval is contingent on the extent to which he feels the acceptance of the group. If he is rejected by the group but is not aware of the rejection, he may still be able to function as though he were part of it. The identity with the group remains intact even though he has been eased to the periphery.

If, however, he is aware of the rejection of the group, or at least believes he is being rejected, he is placed in a painful dilemma. To remain with the group under these circumstances would stimulate considerable lowering of self-esteem. He could then either persist in his efforts to identify with the group and live with the resulting feeling of devaluation, or he could seek identity with another group that would be less satisfying but would at least be available.

Thus, in a passive and gradual manner he drifts into a relationship with the new group. He finds it easier to change his identification than to attempt to overcome the obstacle of resistance he experiences in the group of his original choice. At first he may resent the new group he is being forced to associate with. However, this resentment, as well as identification, changes under the pressure of his need for community. Another person might identify with a new, but less preferable group, not because he has felt rejected by his former group, but because he has experienced something that causes him to feel less worthy. His own feelings of inadequacy or devaluation do not allow him any greater expectation than to become involved with what he previously would have considered to be an inferior group. The group may not be all he wanted, but it is all he feels he is entitled to.

As in other defense mechanisms, the individual is not aware of the underlying motivation for the choices he is making. In fact, he may rationalize his actions and insist that he is making a deliberate and logical choice. However, his behavior and many of his comments may belie the clear logic of his assertions. Not having dissociated himself completely from his past identifications, he is in conflict between them and the new ones he is attempting to establish. This is particularly true during the period of transition following the loss of sight. It is during this period that he can be helped most effectively to consider the meaning of his choices and the available alternatives.

Very frequently, persons who have lost their sight or are in the process of losing it are struggling with this problem of identification. They attempt to maintain their former identification in spite of their loss of sight, or they give in and take on identification with a new group known as "the blind." The critical point on which the struggle hinges is the loss of sight and its accompanying feelings of devaluation.

IDENTIFICATION WITH THE SIGHTED

Some individuals who lose their sight attempt, against all opposition, to maintain their identification with the sighted. They avoid all contacts with other blind persons because of the possible implications that they are members of "the blind." They go to extreme lengths to give the appearance of being sighted. This is particularly true of a person who retains minimal sight. Through his behavior he will attempt to convey the impression that he is able to see more than he actually can. In a doctor's office he pretends to read a magazine when, to him, the print is only a meaningless blur. He pretends to watch a scene outside of a window when, in fact, he can see little beyond the pane of glass. This is not to say that a person with visual impairment should deliberately assume "blind" behavior, but persons in this group exaggerate their behavior in order to prove they are not blind. A sighted person is supposed to function or behave in certain ways, and the visually impaired person maintains his identification by behaving in a similar way. Through his behavior he struggles to maintain this image of himself as a sighted person.

In his struggle to maintain this self-concept he has confused the real issue by placing the emphasis on the value of sight, rather than on his worth as a person with or without sight. He has focused on a physical sense rather than on the more meaningful factors such as values, attitudes, and personality, that truly identify him with specific groups.

Often such a person assumes a very critical attitude toward other blind individuals. He may be more condemning or judgmental in this appraisal than a sighted person would be. Because of his exaggerated need to identify with the sighted, he judges other visually impaired persons as he assumes sighted individuals would. The emotional basis for such an attitude is the extreme importance he places on his identification with the sighted. By harshly criticizing others who are visually impaired he feels he is more sighted than the sighted. He has removed himself one additional step from any association with the blind.

Such a person greatly resents any attempt on the part of sighted friends to force him into a contact with another blind person. Blindness or visual impairment, to him, is degrading and the association with another blind person therefore is demeaning. Of course, if he were confronted with such an interpretation, he would deny it indignantly. Only through psychotherapy can he understand the basis for his behavior. Another explanation for such a person's avoidance of other blind persons is that their presence threatens his position in the sighted group. It is as though he thinks of himself as the favored child and when another blind person comes into the group, he sees him as a rival.

Others who identify with sighted persons are those who will deliberately accentuate their blindness in order to be part of a sighted group. They passively accept all help whether they need it or not. They may even take on the stereotyped behavior that is often associated with blindness in the minds of many people. They ingratiate themselves in any way they can and, in a sense, become mascots or wards of the group. Even though they take an inferior role, they gain some self-esteem because of their special status in the group. They have achieved their goal, which is identity with the group they consider to be superior.

IDENTIFICATION WITH THE BLIND

Other blind or partially sighted persons identify solely with those who are visually impaired. They prefer to attend blind agencies or meet with other blind for social activities. They avoid social contacts with sighted persons or groups. If they occasionally attend some social function with sighted persons, the interaction is on a superficial level. They do not feel at ease with those who are sighted and are frequently on their guard when they find it necessary to deal with them. The terminology they employ often expresses their feelings. "Sighted people just don't understand blind people. They mean well, but only another blind person can know." Expressions such as these demonstrate the gap that they feel exists between themselves and sighted groups, and indicate their identification with "their own kind."

There are a number of reasons why blind persons identify with blind groups. They may have hostile feelings toward those who still can see. They may have had an unfortunate experience with some sighted person and from this experience generalize to all the sighted. A more common reason for the change of identification from a sighted group to a blind group is the devaluation that a person experiences following the loss of sight. Such a person is all too conscious of the many things he can no longer do, especially during the early stages of visual loss. He may have felt inadequate prior to his loss of sight, but now he attributes all his feelings of inadequacy to his loss. Blindness is the cause of his lowered self-esteem and his inferior status. "And because I am blind, I belong with others who have the same affliction." Some visually impaired persons who identify with a blind group minimize the value or degree of their remaining vision. They assume the behavior of someone who cannot see at all. They eagerly solicit help when they do not need it and pretend clumsiness when walking with someone who can see. They deliberately avoid letting other blind persons know the extent of their remaining sight. If they discuss it at all within a group of blind individuals, they describe their sight in terms of how little they have left rather than how much remains.

It is true, of course, that they do have limited sight. They would be restricted in their ability to function even if they used their remaining vision effectively. They are, in fact, exaggerating their limitations rather than completely misrepresenting them. Their behavior is a means of maintaining identity with a group of which they have become a part. Because of their lowered self-esteem, they feel at home with other blind persons, many of whom actually have less sight than they do. Having found security, it is essential to their feeling of well being to be identified with the group.

If they function as though totally blind, it is because they fear that those with less sight might resent — and possibly reject — them. Unless they are part of the group with which they identified themselves, they feel the devastating effects of alienation.

APPROPRIATE IDENTIFICATION

The visually impaired person who does not identify with a group because its members are blind or sighted uses the mechanism more appropriately. He feels comfortable in whichever group he happens to be. He neither avoids nor seeks out a person on the basis of a physical ability but rather on the basis of political, religious, or other values. He feels kinship with those in his own profession or occupation, and identifies with those who have similar recreational interests. The relevant or determining factor for him is the values of a particular group, rather than a physical characteristic or lack of it. Through such identification, he derives greater meaning and satisfaction from his relationships.

CHAPTER 19

COMPENSATION AND OVER-COMPENSATION

The mechanism of compensation is a means of substituting something for what has been lost. It may be a position of favor with a significant person or the actual loss of a treasured object. On the other hand, it may be the loss of a body part — such as a limb — through amputation, or one of the senses — such as seeing or hearing — through impairment.

DEVELOPMENT OF COMPENSATION

The mechanism of compensation appears in the normal process of growth and development during childhood. Initially, the child is helpless and dependent. He requires the nurturance and protection of his parents in order to survive. As he grows, however, he acquires various skills as well as the ability to care for himself. The satisfaction he derives from his increased feeling of independence is compensation or a substitute for the nurturance he once received. Similarly, the increased status he may experience as he becomes more "grown up" is compensation for his replacement by a younger sibling. He feels compensated if he receives privileges that the younger sibling does not have.

In this way the compensation mechanism begins and develops. Eventually it becomes a means of dealing with the normal discouragements and disappointments of life. By concentrating or focusing on compensating factors, the person minimizes the emotional pain or injury he feels following what

he interprets as a loss. The appropriate use of this mechanism
does not mean that the person has to believe that what he lost
was not worthwhile. He can still feel or know that what he lost
had some value. What it does mean is that he faces the loss, but
knows that he can substitute something that has its own worth
for what he has lost. He need not disparage what he lost, but
can appreciate and develop whatever is available as a replacement.

This mechanism is especially useful when attempting to deal
with something as serious as the loss of sight. The individual
need not take the sour grapes attitude: "My sight was not very
important." He can admit that his sight was precious and
valuable and that the loss was painful. But he can also realize
that by developing other traits, skills, or qualities, he can
compensate for his loss. He can work to improve the efficiency
of his other senses; he can retrain and find a new career or
recreation. And he can come to the realization that his worth as
an individual is not based on the presence or absence of sight,
but rather on what he is or can become as a person.

THE EFFECTS OF COMPENSATION

If compensation is a dominant reaction to difficult life
situations, then it certainly will be evident in the process of
adjustment to the loss of sight. It will not prevent the appearance of the various features of emotional reaction stemming
from the loss of sight. It will, however, facilitate the resolution
of the feelings that are a necessary part of the process culminating in eventual adjustment or emotional equilibrium. The
devaluation that the person experiences following his loss will
gradually be replaced by a return to appropriate self-esteem. In
time, the individual will realize that he is not less of a person
because he has lost his sight. He will feel different as he learns
to function by methods other than his former reliance on sight.
But he knows that his reliance on new methods for daily
functioning make him no less worthwhile than he was prior to
his loss.

Anxiety decreases as he discovers that he can cope with
problems and obstacles he once thought were insurmountable. He compensates for his lost sight by acquiring skills that
help him to perform household tasks or to travel to and from

work. By learning to travel with the use of a cane or a guide dog, he has found another way to meet his traveling needs.

If he has lost his job and is still of an employable age, he may retrain and again become employed. He may even compensate to the extent of returning to college, obtaining a degree, and changing his occupation completely. He might even embark on a career that once would have been beyond his aspirations. Any or all of these may be at his disposal to restore damaged self-image. However, what he does in the process of compensation is not nearly as important as how he interprets it. If he interprets what he is able to do as adequate replacement for his lost sight, then he is, in fact, compensating. If, however, he does not, then he still may feel cheated and dissatisfied in spite of his accomplishments following the loss of sight. In such a case the mechanism of compensation is not functioning.

OVER-COMPENSATION

The mechanism of over-compensation functions in a manner similar to that of compensation. However, the individual's response is exaggerated. He gives the impression that he is not simply replacing something he has lost, but that he is attempting to become something more than he was prior to the loss. He seems to be trying to prove to himself and to others that he is a normal and worthwhile person, but his actions indicate that he does not really believe this.

In his effort to demonstrate his worth he makes almost superhuman attempts to cover his apparant deficiencies. He is not satisfied simply to be an adequate blind or visually impaired person. He must show that he is better than any sighted person. In his efforts to retain his former self-image, he attempts to do things that are at best impractical and at worst dangerous. For example, he may refuse to carry a cane when he cannot travel safely with his limited sight. He may decide on a career or job that is unsuitable, considering his physical limitations. For example, he may want to become a printer even though his sight is so restricted that he can read only with difficulty. Without being aware of his motivation, he selects this trade as a goal because it is a trade for a sighted person.

The high school student with very limited vision may attempt to play football when he can hardly see other players on the field, risking serious injury. His courage may seem admirable to others, but his motivation is to prove something to himself that he does not feel or believe. A certain element of denial in the individual is required if this mechanism is to work. The visually impaired person may deny that his sight is as bad as, in fact, it is. Even if he is totally blind, he may deny the reality of his physical limitations. Thus, he sets goals for himself that are beyond his real abilities.

I do not wish to leave the impression that all job and task possibilities have been fully and carefully explored. In fact, many tasks or jobs that, at first glance, would seem to be impossible for a blind or visually handicapped person are actually possible. Sometimes only a slight modification of a tool or a machine is all that is necessary to permit a blind person to function on a job. Another consideration is the wide range of ability among those who make up the blind or visually impaired population.

The question of whether or not a person is using the mechanism of over-compensation must be determined by an objective evaluation of his goals and how he interprets his abilities. One person may be able to perform a particular job because he retains some sight. Another person may be able to perform on a job because he is more intelligent or has mechanical aptitude. However, if the person does not have the qualifications or the ability to perform the job, his choice is based on a need to over-compensate for the loss of sight.

The basis for the mechanism of over-compensation may lie in the extreme devaluation a person feels following his loss. The less worthwhile the individual feels, the more extremely he may react to these feelings. Over-compensation may be the only way he can retain a shred of self-esteem. The individual rarely is aware that his actions are unreasonable or counter-productive. All he knows is what he feels about himself and that he wants to regain his self-esteem. Unfortunately, the person who uses this mechanism often gets into situations that guarantee failure. The result is further devaluation. If he sets goals that are certain to result in failure, he can only confirm the feelings of devaluation he has already experienced.

CHAPTER 20

HOPE AND THE PROCESS OF ADJUSTMENT

Some time ago I attended a lecture for visually impaired persons describing the services offered by a well-known eye clinic. During the discussion that followed, I listened with interest to the questions directed to the speaker. At least half the questions requested information on recent developments in the field of ophthalmology.

"Has there been any breakthough in the treatment of glaucoma?" "Is there any new information regarding diabetic retinopathy?" "Do you expect a breakthrough in the treatment of hereditary eye conditions?" The underlying, but unasked question was, "What can medical science do to restore my sight?" Or, in other words, "Is there any hope that I'll see again?"

HOPE AS A MOTIVATING FACTOR

It seems to be a generally accepted belief that hope is an important element in the adjustment to difficult life circumstances and to recovery from physical illness. If a person believes things will be better, he will work toward that end. If he believes he can regain his health, he will mobilize all his energies to achieve that goal. If he has no hope for improvement, he gives up. He does not look for work when he loses his job; he doesn't try to replace the important person in his life when he loses that person through death or abandonment. He doesn't believe he will get well, so he turns his face to the wall and passively waits for the end.

HOPE AND ADJUSTMENT TO THE LOSS OF SIGHT

How does hope affect the process of adjustment to the loss of sight? It is still an essential element in this process. But if it is to have a beneficial effect, it must be directed toward an achievable goal. If the hope is for the recovery of sight when the medical condition is irreversible, it can only interfere with the process of adjustment.

All too often the person who strongly believes he will see again is unwilling to retrain in order to become independent. When he believes his condition is only temporary, he can see no need to subject himself to the ordeal of developing his other senses, or of acquiring necessary skills. Why should he learn to travel with a cane or learn to read braille when he is sure it is only a matter of time until he sees again? Furthermore, he has no need to mourn his lost sight or to become depressed when he is sure he will eventually regain what he has lost. In this way the strong hope for recovery interferes with the normal process of emotional adjustment to a serious loss. This relationship between hope for recovery and motivation for adjustment can be stated as a proposition. The greater the reliance on hope for recovery from loss of sight, the lesser will be the motivation to engage in the rehabilitation process. It is not easy to become involved in the process of rehabilitation and the effort will not seem worthwhile as long as person believes God, will power, or medical science will give him back his sight. A corollary to this proposition is that the degree to which reality is unacceptable is the degree to which hope for recovery will be fostered. In the case of severe visual impairment, this means that the more difficult it is to live without sight, the more important it will be to believe "I will see again."

Other factors, of course, modify these relationships. Family members, friends, or effective counseling can influence a person to begin in a rehabilitation program in spite of strong hope for recovery. In time, the reality of life without sight may not seem to be as unacceptable. Years of living with unfulfilled hope may diminish the reliance on a belief that never seems to materialize. But in the process, the person may waste years of valuable time—years during which he might have built a new and useful life for himself.

It is, of course, possible that some persons might foster hope for recovery and at the same time enter a program of rehabilitation. They hope they will see again, but function as though this won't happen. Instead of sitting and waiting for the fruition of hope, they go about the business of learning to live with visual impairment because this is the way things are right now. In such cases, hope has not interfered with adjustment to visual loss. Rather, it has been compartmentalized as a dream or fantasy that can lend support through a difficult period of life. Such an integration of hope for recovery and active involvement in retraining is, however, unusual. The more common outcome is that hope for recovery interferes with the process of adaptation.

HOPE FOR A FULL AND USEFUL LIFE

Although unwarranted hope for recovery from loss of sight usually interferes with the process of adjustment, hope is still an important motivating force for the visually impaired person. He may be forced to accept the fact that his medical condition is irreversible, but he need not accept the belief that his useful life is over. He no longer has his sight, but he has a potential for activity and for relative independence. With help, he can retrain his other senses. As he acquires compensatory skills, he can regain some of his former independence. He can develop ways of interacting comfortably with others so that his visual impairment does not interfere with his relationships. Through counseling or psychotherapy he can resolve his feelings of loss and regain his self-confidence. Gradually he can develop a new image of himself as an adequate visually impaired person. In this process, hope is an important asset — not as an expectation of seeing again, but as a belief that things will be better.

It is this hope that will support the visually impaired person as he attempts to cope with the problems of adaptation. Gradually he becomes aware that he can learn to do things he at first thought were impossible. He lives with the expectation that he still can have meaningful relationships, and that in spite of a visual handicap he can live a reasonably normal life. It is this hope that will assist the person who is attempting to struggle with the problem of adjusting to the loss of sight. It is a hope that can be fulfilled because it is based on the way things are and not on the way we would like them to be.

CHAPTER 21

HUMOR IN THE PROCESS
OF ADJUSTMENT

Humor is one means of dealing with harsh reality. It is, in a sense, a way of dealing indirectly with a fact that cannot be dealt with openly. Any fact that is painful, embarrassing, or awkward can often be managed by joking about it or by verbalizing it in some other fashion. If you can joke about a serious event, you can cushion its emotional impact.

The use of humor as a means of coping with harsh reality is not necessarily undesirable. It can be a tool for initiating and facilitating the process of adjustment. It can be a tentative reaching out toward a solution. However, when it is used as a way of avoiding a true confrontation with reality, it can interfere with the adaptive process. It can either delay an appropriate resolution of the feelings stemming from a painful experience or it can prevent such a resolution from ever taking place.

Many persons believe that when a visually impaired person uses humor when talking about himself or his condition, it is an indication that he has accepted what has happened to him. They believe that if he can joke about his handicap, he has learned to live with it. Although this may be a reasonable assumption, it may also be far from an accurate assessment of the person's feelings concerning his condition. He may, in fact, be using wit or humor as a defense, or he may be using it as a way of expressing hostility. On the other hand, it may be just what it seems to be — a demonstration that he has made an

137

appropriate adjustment to his condition. Such a person can also use humorous comments to put sighted persons at ease.

For this reason it is important to consider critically the way in which a handicapped person uses humor. If taken at face value, it can be misleading. But if the humor is considered in terms of its content and the meaning behind it, it can be a valuable tool in evaluating the quality of a person's adjustment to his handicap.

HUMOR AS A DEFENSE

Humor is often used as a defense against the feelings stemming from the loss of sight. In such cases the visually impaired person does not wish to discuss a painful experience seriously, so he refers to it humorously. He draws attention away from his feelings by deliberately focusing on the condition. However, because he feels too uncomfortable with the condition to discuss it seriously, he refers to it in a light, humorous manner. He cannot state simply, "I'm blind," or "I'm visually handicapped." He must make the statement in a way intended to elicit a smile. "It's not that I'm blind, it's just that I can't see."

The person who functions with a denial mechanism hides his true feelings, not only from others, but from himself. He speaks flippantly and convinces himself that what he has lost is not important, or at least, does not bother him. He can discuss his experiences as though it were someone else's, and can joke about it because his true feelings are not easily accessible to consciousness. And the feelings that do not come to the surface are relieved of their emotional charge because he refers to them as lightly as possible. In this way he minimizes their potential effect. By joking he tries to demonstrate that what he has lost is not valuable.

Frequently, a visually impaired person will apply a derogatory term to himself as anticipatory response. He might say, "I'm just a blink," or "Just call me blinky." Such terms, if expressed without the smile of the speaker, are clearly derogatory. What the visually impaired person is expressing is what he believes the sighted person thinks of him. But he does it in a way intended to take the sting out of the remark.

In addition, such responses also reveal the measure of the

person's lowered self-esteem. He feels devalued — an object of ridicule. And the feelings are expressed in the comments he makes about himself. He might say, "I'm blind as a bat," when he has difficulty performing a task. What he means is that he feels inadequate because of his visual impairment. He pokes fun at himself because of his lowered self-esteem. But because he is able to express the comments humorously, he does not feel as devalued as he would if he had to admit seriously that he feels inadequate.

HUMOR AS AN EXPRESSION OF HOSTILITY

Frequently, humor is used as an expression of hostility. A typical vehicle for this form of humor is the sarcastic comment. One person makes a derogatory remark directed toward or about some other person, and everyone in the group laughs. The remark, however, is intended to degrade or ridicule the object of the remark. But the intent is disguised with a thin veneer of humor to make it acceptable. Another person will tell a story about something that happened to another individual. Everyone laughs because of some incongruous aspect of the happening. However, the event or its description may be quite embarrassing to the person who is the object of attention. Other well known examples of humor-disguised hostility are political cartoon and racial jokes.

The same expression of hostility is often present in the humor used by some blind or visually impaired persons. They feel anger or hostility toward sighted people in general or a family member in particular. However, they cannot express this feeling in a direct attack because they are dependent on these persons. In these circumstances, they make sarcastic remarks toward or about some family member. They describe an incident in which the sighted person made a mistake while leading them, and they intend these remarks to be degrading or embarrassing to the person. However, they select and emphasize humorous aspects of the situation to disguise their true feelings. Their rationalization is that no one can take offense at a description of something funny.

Such humor is often, however, self-defeating, because the person who is the butt of the joke or the focus of the sarcasm may take offense, even if he does not express his resentment openly. The resentful feelings may interfere with the relationship to the point that he avoids the visually impaired person. Because this type of humor is potentially destructive, it is essential that the person using it be made aware of its potential for harm. He should be helped to understand what he is doing and the motives for what he considers to be humor.

The following is a story told by a blind man. "I was crossing a street one day and happened to veer slightly, so that when I reached the other side, I was touching the grass on the parkway. Now I know that there were dogs in the neighborhood, so for obvious reasons I didn't want to step on the grass. While I was trying to find the sidewalk, someone grabbed me by the arm and I heard a woman saying, 'May I help you?' As I was trying to tell her what I wanted, she pulled me until I discovered I was back on the same side of the street I started from."

"I'd like to get to the north side of the street and turn west," I informed her.

"I'm sorry, but I don't know north from south or east from west."

"Well then, I want to go across the street and turn left."

"Now, by this time several other people had gathered and we had a conference right there on the sidewalk. Finally I asked, 'Is there a mailbox on the corner?' When they said there was, I asked them to take me to it and put my hand on it. When they did, I said goodbye and left them standing there talking among themselves. I found out later that the woman was some poor retarded lady who had admired me for a long time and had been dying for the opportunity to help me."

Most audiences, when told this story, would find it quite humorous. They would laugh at certain incongruities in the situation. A blind man needs help, gets it from someone who is mentally retarded and eventually finds his own way with only minimal help from sighted people.

There is, however, an underlying element of hostility in the message. A mentally retarded woman wishes to help a blind man who supposedly is lost. However, she does not have the capacity to provide the help he needs. She demonstrates her ignorance and slow-wittedness in her bungling attempts to help. Eventually he is forced to ask for help from other sighted persons. But he does not rely on them to help him with the street crossing. So he places them in a category with the retarded woman. In the telling, the retarded woman and the other sighted persons have been devalued. His self-esteem has been elevated by demonstrating his own superiority to sighted people. Because he could say goodbye and find his own way, he has had the last laugh.

HUMOR AS AN INDICATION OF ADJUSTMENT

The person who has made an appropriate adjustment to his loss of sight may sometimes use humor in his communication. He has come to terms with this condition and shows it in the way he uses humor. When used in this framework, the humor accurately represents the state of his emotions at this point in his life. He does have a feeling of devaluation, which he needs to disguise, since he has already recovered his self-esteem. Since he is no longer inappropriately dependent, he does not feel anger toward those who still have what he has lost, he does not ridicule them or employ sarcasm in his communication with them. His visual impairment is part of him and he has learned to live with it. As a result, he uses humor as a tool, not a weapon.

When he uses humor, it is because he sees incongruities that are amusing in his circumstances. He can see an unpleasant happening for what it is. But he can also see that a certain combination of circumstances can produce a ridiculous situation. If he had any appreciation for the ridiculous prior to his loss of sight, he will find things he can laugh at as a visually impaired person. And he will feel comfortable sharing the amusing aspects of his experience.

Falling down, in itself, may not be funny. But if he has not been injured, the way in which he fell may be amusing. Knocking over a drink can be embarrassing, but if when grabbing for the falling drink he knocks over something else, and this triggers a chain reaction of fumbles, the whole situation can become ridiculous and amusing in the telling. Whatever the particular situation may be, humor can be an indication of appropriate adjustment. If the visually impaired person has come to terms with his condition, then the humor he uses will be a reflection of his feelings.

HUMOR AS A BRIDGE TO COMMUNICATION

Many sighted persons feel uncomfortable when they first meet a visually impaired or blind person. The experience is unfamiliar to them and they do not know just how to react. They don't know if he needs help, or how to help him — if this is what he needs. They are not even sure how to ask. They are afraid that if they do ask he might be offended. They feel awkward and do not know how to break through the awkwardness of the moment.

Any blind person who is comfortable with his situation and is aware of such feelings can use humor to stimulate comfortable interaction. By speaking lightly about his needs or his condition he can put the sighted person at ease. He puts the facts on a level that facilitates understanding. A serious discussion of his loss might be inappropriate because he and the sighted person do not have a close relationship. Such a discussion might increase the sighted person's feelings of awkwardness. But a humorous comment referring to the visual condition — or a problem caused by the condition — can ease the strain. The comment indicates to the sighted person that the visually impaired person is comfortable with his situation. If he is at ease, the sighted person need not feel uncomfortable. In effect, the humorous comment gives the sighted person permission to be amused at the incongruity of the situation. He can laugh with the blind person and need not have the feeling that he is laughing at him. The blind person bumps against a wall or a piece of furniture and says, "I don't know how this always gets in my way. The other day I was walking down the street and bumped into a telephone pole right in the middle of the sidewalk!" To which one sighted person replied, "Yeah, I was there and I saw it jump right in front of you just as you got there."

In this example the blind person initiates the humor and the sighted person shares in it. The shared humor shows the sighted person that blindness is not a forbidden subject. The blind person who bumped into the wall might feel embarrassed, and the sighted person who observes it might also feel uncomfortable, but the humorous reference to the incident breaks a barrier to communicaton. They do not have to talk seriously about the condition and probably would not feel comfortable in doing so. But they can refer to it humorously. Even avoiding any mention of it would not be entirely satisfactory, because it would still be in the mind of each. Without the freedom to refer to it in some way, it might inhibit their interaction, and interfere with the possibility of better communication.

The humorous reference to the incident by the blind person, however, removes some of the emotional charge. By verbalizing it in this way the visually impaired person has minimized whatever embarrassment each might feel. So humor has become a way of bridging the distance of blindness between two people. They feel more comfortable in their communication and both can benefit.

SECTION V

TREATMENT

CHAPTER 22

A HOLISTIC APPROACH
TO REHABILITATION

Effective therapy for the person who has lost a major portion of his sight must incorporate both physical retraining and psychological reconstitution. The loss of any major sense necessitates compensatory training of the other senses and acquisition of new skills in order to achieve good functioning. It is only through a holistic approach in therapy that the person will receive adequate help. He is both a physical and a psychological being, and no rehabilitation program which emphasizes one aspect of the individual while ignoring the other can be successful.

The person's ability to function is affected by what he feels about himself and his condition. He may make some gains through physical retraining, but if he has not resolved his feelings about what has happened to him, it is quite possible that he will not use what he has learned. He can complete an entire training course for traveling, but if he is not able to cope with his feelings of anxiety or self-consciousness, he will, in all likelihood, put away the cane and depend on sighted help when he needs to travel. If he cannot get sighted help, he may withdraw completely from social contacts. In a similar way, he may undertake a course in reading and writing braille, and because this symbolizes what he has lost, he may put away his braille books and forget everything he has learned.

Conversely, if he is given only psychological help without being given the physical retraining to restore his independence and self confidence, he can never feel that he is an adequate

147

individual. If he never learns to travel without help and if some other person meets every need, he cannot feel that he is a productive individual. Furthermore when an agency offers only arts and crafts courses to a visually impaired person, it confirms his feelings of devaluation. The visually impaired person compares the activity in which he is encouraged to participate, with the activity he enjoyed prior to his loss of sight. By comparison, the simplicity of his present activity demonstrates undeniably that he is no longer the capable person he once was.

Of course, if the tasks he is expected to perform are only preliminary to the performance of more complex tasks that will ultimately lead to useful and productive activity, they can serve a useful purpose. They can be an integral part of the rehabilitation. However, they cannot be an end in themselves if they are to have a rehabilitative function. If the total rehabilitation program includes both physical retraining and emotional adjustment, the person eventually realizes that he is still a useful and worthwhile person. He finds that he can perform tasks that he once thought were beyond his ability. In addition, he resolves the feelings of loss and adapts emotionally to his new situation.

Some agencies have taken a holistic approach to the problem and provide a comprehensive program for their clients. All too often, however, agency administrators take a narrow view of the problem and provide only physical retraining. They provide only those services that seem to have an immediate and visible result. Adequate studies might indicate that this short sighted view does not give long term benefits.

Often, programs are initiated in a haphazard fashion. Services are added or turned down on the basis of what other agencies are offering; or they are restricted because of the cost, although the service might be beneficial to the client. There is sufficient evidence in the literature to demonstrate that any successful rehabilitative effort must be directed toward the whole person. Emotional needs are just as real as physical needs. This is true whether the condition is visual impairment or some other handicap. No matter what blow a person has suffered, he will react emotionally to the physical condition. We are not simply physical beings — automatons; we are emotional beings as well. We have feelings and thoughts about everything that happens to us.

CHAPTER 23

THE ROLE OF THE PHYSICIAN

When an individual has lost or is in the process of losing his sight, the ophthalmologist, by virtue of his professional status, will have a significant impact on the patient's adjustment to the loss. This aspect of the role of the physician is, of course, secondary to his primary role which is the treatment and cure of disease and injury. He may be treating the patient when the fact of blindness becomes inescapable or he may be examining him in his role as a consultant. In either case, his interaction with the patient is crucial because he is the medical expert, and because the patient may be at a critical point in his medical history.

At this point, the patient undoubtedly has some awareness of the seriousness of his condition. He may not verbalize his hopes and fears, but they are present. If his condition is progressive, he may have been observing changes with almost obsessive concern. From one day to the next he will watch for even minute differences in his visual ability. He will certainly react to each reduction in sight with apprehension, but also, with hope for a cure.

Although hope for recovery may be essential in other medical conditions, in the case of blindness, it may actually interfere with the adjustment process. The patient must have a realistic evaluation of his condition before he can begin to make an adjustment. It is the role of the physician to release the patient from false hope that will interfere with his complete use of available rehabilitation services. Honesty and frankness are imperative insofar as the diagnosis and prognosis permit. If a patient is told that he will never go blind, and his vision continues to deteriorate, inevitably he will lose confidence in his doctor.

One older woman phrased it this way: "I have diabetic retinopathy, and when I first started losing the sight in one eye, the doctor said it would not happen to my other eye. Now I'm losing sight in that eye and he says I won't go completely blind, but I'll never believe anything he tells me again."

If the prognosis is, in fact, uncertain, or if the condition is irreversible, the patient has the right to know this. When he knows, he can begin to deal with the reality as he will experience it. He is then free to proceed through the emotional reaction to his loss and make the fullest use of his remaining assets and abilities.

It may seem a kindness to permit the patient to believe that he will never go completely blind or that a cure may be possible some day. However, anxiety concerning an uncertain condition can be as stressful as certain knowledge of a loss. It may, in fact, be more destructive, and ultimately contrary to the best interests of the patient. In addition, it may encourage the patient to retain unrealistic goals. He may thus lose valuable time and emotional energy that could be spent better in the work of successful rehabilitation.

If a patient has had prior treatment or examination, he may have had some knowledge of his condition. If he is being informed for the first time concerning his condition, he may experience a period of stress or crisis. In either case, the doctor is in a prime position to make the appropriate referral, whether this is for counseling, psychotherapy, or a rehabilitation agency.

If the patient has just been faced with the reality of his condition, he may need a few days to begin absorbing the meaning of the information he has received. However, according to crisis intervention theory, it is during such a period of crisis that his defenses are down, and he may be more ready to accept help then he would at a later time. For this reason, it is imperative that he be referred for therapy while he is in this crisis state.

Occasionally a patient may express anger or resentment toward the doctor. The feelings may be completely unrelated to the medical facts. They may be a reaction to the blow dealt by an unkind fate. Thus, the patient verbally lashes out at whomever happens to be available. These angry feelings also may be a reaction to the patient's own feelings of guilt because of his procrastination in seeking medical help. The reaction is irrational and unjustified, but it serves as a release.

The manner of presenting information to the patient is extremely important. It can be realistic and still have the element of compassion and kindness. It can be candid and accurate without being brutal or harsh. It need not imply pity on the doctor's part. It can be of value to the patient just to know that the doctor is aware that the loss of sight is a severe blow, that many visual experiences are no longer possible or are severely restricted.

Although some emphasis can be placed on the patient's abilities or potential, it is doubtful that he will grasp all of this information while he is still trying to deal with the full impact of the loss. However, such an emphasis can set the direction for the patient. It can point to hope for a full life, and not to hope for recovery — a false hope that the patient ultimately will question, no matter what information he receives.

CHAPTER 24

REFERRALS AND RESISTANCE TO REHABILITATION

Once a person who has lost his sight has been told that his condition is irreversible, he should be referred to those best qualified to help him. It is unlikely that such a person can rapidly and effectively rehabilitate himself, since few people have adequate knowledge of just what is involved in the process of adaptation to severe loss of sight. In most cases, the needs of such persons are varied and they require help from more than one source. Where some sight remains, every consideration should be given to the possibility that it may be enhanced through the use of visual aids or special devices such as closed circuit television. The patient should be directed to a low vision clinic or to some professional specializing in this area. Some persons have lost their income and need help from a social welfare agency that can restore at least a minimal income. Others need vocational guidance since they can no longer function in their former occupation. Certainly when a person has lost a drastic amount of sight, he requires retraining in physical skills to compensate for his visual loss. Above all, the need for psychotherapy or counseling should not be overlooked. It can be the foundation for total rehabilitation.

Whatever the special needs of the person who has lost his sight, it is imperative that he be put in touch with the source best able to meet his needs. One client informed me that it took him almost a year to get adequate information concerning agencies that could provide the help he needed. He was particularly bitter because he had spent two weeks in a hospital following his loss of sight, and felt that during this tme he should have been given information that would have shortened his period of rehabilitation.

RESISTANCE TO REHABILITATION

One might assume that anyone losing a major portion of his sight would want to be rehabilitated. Such a person must be aware of his limitations. How can he travel, work, take care of his everyday needs, or cope with his feelings? Who will train him? Where can he get information? All he needs is someone to tell him where to go or give him a telephone number to call. It's simple. And, of course, many persons accept the referral and get the help and training they need. But there are others who resist any attempt to give them help or information. You tell them, "Go to this place," or "Call this number," and they say, "I'm not interested," or "I'm not ready yet," or "I don't need it. No one can help me." They may resist in a passive manner. They take the address or phone number with thanks, but when you next see them they have done nothing to make a contact. "I haven't gotten around to it yet," or "I don't have any way of getting there." The would-be helper feels frustrated. He sees that the visually impaired person is not managing well, but because of the resistance, he feels as though he is pushing against a stone wall.

But the person may also seem to accept the referral. He goes to the agency and signs up for classes, but makes little progress as a student. His attendance is irregular. He misses special appointments with staff members. He doesn't do assignments — or does them haphazardly. If he makes any progress, it is far below his intellectual or physical ability. A staff member suggests that a course such as braille or mobility training will help him, and he argues that nothing can help or he will never use it. He can get help "some other way." Training that he should complete in six months drags on interminably. He says he wants to learn but he doesn't. He becomes a perennial student at an agency and does little to help himself. His behavior pattern shows he is resistant to rehabilitation.

The reason for it may be complicated and not readily

apparent. Many persons feel they are giving up hope if they contact any agency serving the blind. They cling to the belief they will see again and convince themselves they do not need help with their blindness. They can maintain this belief only by staying away from any agency concerned with rehabilitation. Their resistance is directed against the thought of giving up hope for recovery. Others make the first contact but are overwhelmed by the presence of so many blind persons in one place. Suddenly they are confronted by the knowledge that they are members of this group. They have come once but wish only to escape. One man in his early thirties who had been to an agency twice told me he cried each time, thinking about all those blind people. Such feelings are especially prevalent among those who have not lost all their sight. They think of everyone around them as being totally blind and helpless, and expect this will happen to them eventually. Their only thought is to get away from any reminder of what they fear.

Anxiety may be the main reason visually impaired individuals resist attempts to provide help. In their own home they can manage, but the thought of going somewhere new and finding their way around unfamiliar buildings frightens them. It also occurs to them that most of the people they will meet are blind, so how can they get help? And if all their life they have used sight to learn things, how can they learn now when they can no longer see and read?

Some may resist rehabilitation because they are self-conscious. "Doesn't everyone there have to use a white cane? I'm not ready for that yet." Or, "My friends will want to know where I'm going and I'm not ready to tell them it's a place for the blind." Family pressure is another basis for the visually impaired person's resistance. Various family members encourage him to believe he will see again. They are not ready to admit the finality of his blindness. "So why get into a rehabilitation program now? Maybe you won't need it. Besides, we can give all the help you need. We'll guide you by the hand, but if you carry a white cane, people will stare."

Such pressure may be all it takes to solidify resistance when a person is vacillating between getting help and running away from the problem. He will take the easy way and remain at home, depending on family members to meet his needs.

These same factors may be present for those persons who re-

sist during the course of training. A student may be going
through the motions but is afraid. He may not say, "I won't do
it," but is reluctant because of anxiety. He does not learn well or
avoids assignments because he is tense and afraid. He thinks he
may be injured if he attempts to travel or cook a meal. So he
does nothing and makes excuses. The self-conscious person
also may avoid assignments but does so because someone may
see him make a mistake. He feels awkward if he stumbles or
when he misses the container when he pours liquid into a cup.
Rather than give an explanation, he resists the instructor's
efforts to help. Often such resistance is complicated by family
members who remind the visually impaired person that he can
be hurt or that he looks clumsy when he makes a mistake. Instead of encouraging him, they undermine the little motivation
he has. They tell him, "I'm willing to help. Isn't that good
enough?" And so, rather than displease the person on whom he
is dependent, he becomes resistant in training.

Frequently a very simple basis for resistance is the lack of information. The person says, "You can't help me," because he
does not know what kind of help the rehabilitation agency
offers. He is aware of his limitations but does not know there
are specific courses to help him acquire new skills. He does not
know that even a totally blind person can learn to travel independently. Or that there are special devices and techniques
which will help him to perform daily tasks. He may not know
that he can be retrained to work and that there are laws to aid
the physically handicapped. When it is evident that there is
resistance in a client, one must deal with it. It is not enough to
describe him as being resistant to rehabilitation, nor will it accomplish anything to give him a pep talk. Instead, he should be
referred to a counselor — someone who understands his
feelings and knows his potential in a rehabilitation program.
Occasionally a friend or family member will contact an agency
concerning someone who says he does not want help. It is possible to convince such a person in a phone conversation to
come in for just one counseling session without committing
himself to enroll or even return for an additional session. In
that session it may be possible to deal with his resistance. But
where there has been such an agreement, it is important not to
pressure the client into any further commitment or it will in-

crease his resistance. He should be given the freedom to return or not as he chooses.

When there is resistance during training, it is also important to determine the basis for the behavior rather than simply dismissing him as being a difficult student. Sometimes an instructor can help a student overcome the resistance if he knows the student is afraid or that there is family interference. In most cases, however, it is advisable to refer the client for counseling in order to help him resolve his feelings. When family members contribute to the resistance, it is helpful to provide counseling for them, also. Only by dealing with resistance can the visually impaired person benefit from the help available to him at a rehabilitation agency.

CHAPTER 25

CRISIS INTERVENTION
AND GROUP COUNSELING

The principles of crisis intervention therapy are applicable when the loss of sight is sudden and drastic, or when the medical condition stabilizes after the initial loss. With professional help it is sometimes possible for such a person to resolve his feelings within a period of weeks.

Statistics indicate that many persons in lower socio-economic groups return for only two or three counseling sessions. When it is evident that the person who has lost his sight is in this category, it is imperative that the therapist intervene actively for the few sessions available to him. Such intervention is also essential when the client has a limited education and finds it difficult to verbalize his feelings.[2] Of course, it should be conducted judiciously since these persons are often resistant and intervention that is too active might increase their resistance.

An additional argument for such therapy is that many persons do not apply for rehabilitation services when they first lose their sight. They may not have been referred by their ophthalmologist or they may have resisted the suggestion that they apply for services. Thus, when they finally reach out for help, they have lived for years as poorly functioning blind persons. During this time, they have developed self-defeating patterns of behavior and lowered self-esteem. Helping them achieve a healthier self-concept requires considerably longer than if they had made the contact for help while in a state of crisis.

Some persons may seem to function quite well because their

loss of sight is gradual. But even they may require some therapy during the period in which a critical change is taking place. For example, when a person can no longer drive or read a newspaper, he finds it difficult to avoid facing the fact of his loss.

When the loss is progressive, the actual difference in visual acuity may seem small to the observer. But to the person with little sight, even a minute degree of loss takes on great significance. In fact, the less sight the person retains, the more aware he will be of each tiny reduction. Because he has so little, he will feel each successive loss acutely.

One percent loss is probably not significant to a person with twenty-twenty vision, but a one percent loss to the person with only three percent of normal sight is a drastic change which can be frightening. Not only does this loss further restrict his ability to function, but it represents another step in the direction of total blindness. It represents a defeat in the sense that his hope has not been justified or that his fears have been confirmed.

Many individuals in this group are quite willing and able to discuss their feelings and experience in therapy, and benefit greatly. However, each client must be considered as an individual rather than as a member of a group. Furthermore, the therapist must be sensitive to the responses of the client and maintain a balance between active intervention and stimulation of resistance.

LIMITATIONS OF CRISIS INTERVENTION

Two factors that limit the efficacy of crisis intervention are the personality of the patient and the progress of the visual loss. If the loss of sight exacerbates already existing psychic disturbances, then, of course, short term counseling will not suffice. The person may be just within his ability to cope and the added stress of visual loss may precipitate a breakdown. In this case, it may take months or years to resolve the feelings resulting from the loss of sight.

When the loss of sight occurs over a long period of time, such as months or years, it is unrealistic to assume that accompanying feelings can be easily resolved. This is equally true when the condition is unstable: deterioration followed by stability or slight recovery, followed by further loss. In fact, the patient will experience numerous crises. Each successive reduction will stimulate further anxiety and each stable period will stir up hope that no further loss will occur. Each minute change is a signal of what could happen to him, and each time he must adjust to the change. It is imperative that such a person be given longer term supportive therapy. If he is terminated from counseling while his visual loss is still in progress, he will have a valid reason for interpreting the termination as abandonment. Some persons are so resistant to the idea of attending an agency for the blind that they refuse even to make a contact.

In other cases, the period of adjustment is prolonged because of personality conflicts, the rigidity of defenses, or the special meaning of blindness to the individual. It would be unrealistic to assume that, in such cases, short term therapy could greatly benefit the client.

GROUP COUNSELING

Group counseling is another tool that can be useful in helping an individual to resolve the feelings and problems stemming from the loss of sight. It has certain benefits, but it also has limitations. For this reason, it should never be the automatic treatment when a person loses his sight. Each person must be considered for group counseling in terms of his special problems and needs. In addition, he must be evaluated with regard to emotional readiness for a group experience before he is assigned to a group.

One important benefit the individual can derive from group counseling is the opportunity to vent his feelings to others. In other words, he can say what he feels in a semi-structured social situation. As the person expresses his feelings in the group, or listens to others do so, he discovers that his feelings are not unique. He hears others express feelings of anger, bitterness, and resentment. He learns that others feel anxiety and frustration as they attempt to struggle with the problems of everyday life. Not only does he learn that he is not alone in what he feels, but as he cautiously expresses these feelings, he can test for the reaction to what he is saying. If another group member is critical or is indifferent to his comments, he can learn to cope with such reactions. This can be especially helpful if the group leader or other members of the group are supportive, or encourage him as he tries to verbalize his feelings.

During the course of group work, there will be considerable sharing of learning experiences that will benefit most members. One member may describe how he has solved a family problem. Another may tell how he has been able to find a way of performing some task. The person who acquires the new bit of information benefits as he adds to his store of knowledge. The person who explains his particular solution benefits; his self-esteem grows because he has been able to help someone else. To the extent that the members of the group are able to apply what they learn to their interaction with sighted friends or family, they all benefit. Such sharing of information can provide considerable positive reinforcement in the process of adjustment to the loss of sight.

Although group counseling for visually impaired persons has its benefits, it also has its limitations. If the group constantly focuses on problems of visual loss to the exclusion of all other problems, the effect can be detrimental. Visual loss then becomes the basis and the explanation for almost every problem of life. Normal difficulties of social interaction often are excused or explained away in terms of the visual impairment. Failures are often attributed to the visual handicap when, in fact, they may be a function of personality problems.

An additional limitation of group counseling for visually impaired persons is that the group may unite on the basis of their identity with each other in opposition to the sighted public. Their sense of sharing a common problem that is not shared by the larger community can create a climate that is unfavorable to appropriate adjustment. The various members may satisfy their need for security in the group, and as a result, do not feel a need to re-establish relationships in the larger society.

SELECTING GROUP MEMBERS

A primary consideration in selecting persons for group counseling should be the emotional readiness of the individual for the group experience. If a person is severely depressed, the preferable treatment is individual counseling or psychotherapy. The person may be so involved with his own feelings that he cannot benefit from the solutions of others. Furthermore, listening to the difficulties that other members of the group face may depress him even further. In addition, if he overtly and repeatedly expresses the depth of his despair in the group, the other group members might become disturbed by his morbid concentration on his loss.

Individuals can be selected for group counseling on the basis of group goals, such as employment. The discussions can then be structured to include problems of obtaining employment, or employer attitudes toward hiring visually impaired persons.

When some special goal is not the basis for forming a counseling group, there should be an attempt to achieve as much heterogeneity as possible. The group should include both males and females, as well as a fairly wide age range, in order to achieve some balance in discussion. One young person alone in a group of elderly individuals would feel out of place and would have little to discuss when the other members of the group focus on problems of aging and social security benefits. Similarly, one elderly person in a group discussing problems of employment might feel that he cannot interact with the group on any meaningful level.

One group composition that should be considered is a combination of visually impaired, and sighted, but handicapped persons. Such a composition should minimize the possibility that visually impaired persons would focus exclusively on problems relating to their lost sight. The sighted members of the group could benefit from the involvement with persons trying to cope with a different handicap. A further benefit for the visually impaired persons is the opportunity for immediate feedback from sighted persons regarding their special problems and fears. The group could be a bridge between themselves and others in the sighted community. All would benefit as they share similar feelings, although their physical problems might be different. The formation of such a group would require cooperation between agencies serving visually impaired persons and those serving persons with other handicaps. This would provide a fringe benefit for staff members, in giving them wider professional experience working with persons having differing problems.

CHAPTER 26

DOES A PERSON EVER
GET USED TO BEING BLIND?

Does a person ever get used to being blind? This is a question that many people ask, although probably many more never put it into words. It is a question that must be considered because it is implied in the whole process of learning to live with a major handicap. The entire process of adjustment to the loss of sight is no more than an attempt to cope with what has happened. It is a process of getting used to being blind or visually impaired, and we must consider whether such a goal is even possible.

HOW IS THE QUESTION ASKED?

There are many ways of asking or implying the question. Some persons ask quite bluntly, "Have you ever gotten used to being blind?" They speak right out with the thought that occurs to them when they meet a blind person. Others ask less directly, "Does anyone ever get used to being blind?" They are perhaps a little more sensitive to the feelings of the person to whom they direct the question, but they are still sufficiently motivated to ask. Still others ask more obliquely. They dig for information without ever actually putting into words the thing they really want to know. They ask on the periphery of the real issue in hope of discovering what they hesitate to ask openly. "How can you find your way to where you're going?" "Do you travel by yourself?" "How can you eat when you can't see what's on your plate?" "Do blind people ever marry sighted people?" or "Can your wife see?" "Is it hard for a blind person to get dressed by himself?" or "How can you tie your shoes without seeing?"

In each case, the questioner had a definite idea in mind. He wanted to know the true meaning of blindness. He wanted to know if it were possible to live without sight. In other words, "Can a person ever get used to being blind?" Most persons, however, never ask the question. They are interested in the answer, but are too reticent to ask. They wonder, but do not wish to offend the person with a visual impairment.

WHO ASKS THE QUESTION

The persons interested in the matter of learning to live with visual impairment can be placed in four general groups. The ones who are most critically interested are those who have recently lost their sight, or are in the process of losing it. The second group is the family of a person who has lost his sight. Then there are the professionals who work with visually impaired clients. The final group interested in the question is a large segment of the general population.

WHY ASK THE QUESTION

It is readily apparent that the person who has just lost his sight or is losing it has an immediate interest in the question. He wants to know if the feelings he is experiencing will ever dissipate. Will the fear, anger, frustration, or depression that seems to have overwhelmed him be with him for the rest of his life, or can he feel good again? He wants to know if any meaningful life is possible for him without sight. He is asking because he wants to be given some hope.

What the family members want to know is directly related to the outcome for the visually impaired person. They are just as uncertain and confused as he is. The answer to the question is vitally important to them, because their future — their expectations and choices — depends on it.

The professional may have a different reason for asking, but the answer is just as relevant for him. He is interested in the well-being of the patient, and he wants to know if the patient can have a meaningful life. If so, he can help to set realistic and useful goals. As a professional, he wants to use his skills to the best advantage of the patient. The goals he sets must be realistic or his efforts are pointless. He asks because he wants to know if what he is doing is worthwhile.

The motives are less obvious for the majority of persons who ask or think the question. In addition, the reasons for asking are mixed. Each person has an element of curiosity that stirs whenever he sees someone who looks or acts differently from himself. He wants to know how the visually impaired person thinks, feels, and lives. By observation, he can know how the person sounds and acts, but he cannot know how he thinks and feels.

Often, however, the reason for the question is more personal than mere idle curiosity. The real motivation behind the question is another question. "How would I feel if this happened to me? Would I be able to make it? Could I live with it? Or, would I go to pieces? What would life be like if I couldn't see?" Sometimes, such an individual identifies with the blind person, imagining what it would be like to be blind. He would like to believe that if it happened to him, he would "overcome." If he can believe that the blind person will "make it" and have a good life, then he can believe he, himself, will "make it" too.

THE ANSWER

We could answer the question affirmatively and say, "Yes, a person can get used to being blind." Such an answer is true, but it is also misleading. A more honest answer is that some persons get used to being blind and some do not. Part of the problem is in how the question and the answer is defined. If, by "getting used to being blind" a person means the difference between being happy or unhappy, or never having any problems, both the question and the answer are invalid. It would perhaps be more accurate to say that some persons can learn to live with the loss of sight and make the most of what is left, while others cannot. It might, in fact, be helpful to talk about other life circumstances and how people live with them.

There are very few people who, in the course of their life, do not experience some serious loss or blow. For most people, life is simply not a "bowl of cherries"; for some it occasionally is; for many others it never is. Many people spend their entire lives in grinding poverty. They simply exist from one day to the next, and for them the primary problem is one of survival. Many never really feel well, or live for years within the border of unremitting pain.

Crippling as the result of disease or physical injury is a fact of life for many people. This may vary from the loss of one or two fingers or toes to almost total disability. The condition may be only temporary, but in many cases it is permanent and the person is forced to live with a reduced capacity to function.

Most individuals learn to live within their situation, whether this is one of physical limitation or one of economic hardship. If given a choice, they would, in most cases, choose a more comfortable life style. Those with physical limitations would undoubtedly prefer the full use of their physical faculties. They may not be satisfied or pleased with their circumstances, but have within themselves a strong will to survive. And beyond mere survival, they usually have a desire to get the most satisfaction or pleasure that is possible within the restrictions imposed on them. Thus, the person with a physical disability would prefer to be physically normal, but if this is not possible, he will settle for whatever he can get within his means and abilities. This is precisely the basis on which most people who lose their sight come to terms with their limitations. If given a true choice, they would choose to see as well as they ever did. But if second best — visual impairment — is what they must live with, then this is what they do.

In attempting to answer the question, I do not intend to minimize the serious nature of visual impairment. Sight is a valuable sense and the loss of it is a serious blow. The adjustment to life without sight, or with only minimal sight, is a difficult process. However, it is not the end of life, even though it may seem so at the time.

In the loss of sight, as in every difficult or painful experience, life centers around the ability to accept things as they are. We may not enjoy the pain of loss, but we adapt to it. Pain diminishes as the wound heals. It becomes less significant as other things gain in importance. We live with the condition and attempt to get satisfaction from what remains to us.

The process of adaptation takes time, and as members of a human community we need help. Given the time and appropriate help, most persons learn to live with the limitations of visual impairment.

So, in a qualified sense, we answer the question in the affirmative. It *is* possible to get used to being blind. Happiness is *not* being blind; it comes in spite of or apart from the loss of sight. Contentment, pleasure, satisfaction, or whatever criteria we wish to use as a measure of the quality of life, are beyond the simple matter of sight or the lack of it. There is certainly no guarantee that a person will get used to being blind or visually handicapped, but if over a period of time he resigns himself to his condition as a fact of life, he can look forward to making the most of what he has left. He learns whatever is necessary, so he can live as effectively as possible. He accepts himself for what he is, a person with a visual impairment, but also a person with real potential. He learns to exploit this potential, and in the process finds that he can get used to being blind.

FINIS

REFERENCES

1. Blank, Robert. "Psychoanalysis and Blindness." *The Psychoanalytic Quarterly*, Vol. XXVI, no. 1 (1957): 1-23.

2. Capland, Gerald. *A Community Approach to Mental Health.* New York: Grune & Stratton, 1961.

3. Carroll, Thomas J. *Blindness: What It Is, What It Does, and How To Live With It.* Boston: Little, Brown and Company, 1961.

4. Chevigny, Hector, and Braverman, Sydell. *The Adjustment of the Blind.* New York: Yale University Press, 1950.

5. Cholden, Louis, A. *A Psychiatrist Works With Blindness.* New York: American Foundation for the Blind, Inc., 1958.

6. Coleman, James C. *Abnormal Psychology and Modern Life.* Chicago: Scott Foresman Co., 1956.

7. Finestone, Samuel. *Social Casework and Blindnes.* New York: American Foundation for the Blind, 1960.

8. Litman, Robert E., M.D. "Prevention of Suicide." *Current Psychiatric Therapies*, Vol. VI (1966).

9. National Society for the Prevention of Blindness, Inc. *Estimated Statistics on Blindness and Vision Problems.* New York: National Society for the Prevention of Blindness, Inc., 1966.

10. Rochlyn, Gregory, M.D. "The Dread of Abandonment: A Contribution to the Etiology of the Loss Complex and to Depression." *The Psychoanalytic Study of the Child*, Vol. 63, 82-6, 451-69.

11. Schulz, Paul J., "A Group Approach to Working With Families of the Blind." *The New Outlook for the Blind*, Vol. 63, no. 3 (March 1968): 82-86.

12. ——. "The Emotional Reaction to the Loss of Sight." In *Psychiatric Aspects of Ophthalmology*, pp. 38-67. Edited by Adams, Peralman & Sloan. Springfield: Charles C. Thomas, 1974.

13. ——."Psychological Factors in Orientation and Mobility Training." *The New Outlook for the Blind*, Vol. 66, no. 5 (May 1972) 129-34.

14. Scott, Robert A. *The Making of Blind Men.* New York: Russell Sage Foundation, 1969.

15. Stein, Jules. "Eye Research — The Key to Blindness Prevention." *Eye Research Seminar,* (November 1965): 5-7.

16. Ward, Allen L., Ph.D. "The Response of Individuals Beginning Work With Blind Persons." *The New Outlook for the Blind,* Vol. 67, no. 1 (January 1973).

INDEX